JUICING FOR

DIABETES

Fast and Easy Recipe for Weight loss, Body Detox, Eliminate Sugar and

Regulate Blood Pressure

BONUS: FREE RECIPE JOURNAL TO START YOUR

JUICING JOURNEY.

FOR PAPERBACK AND HARDCOVER ONLY.

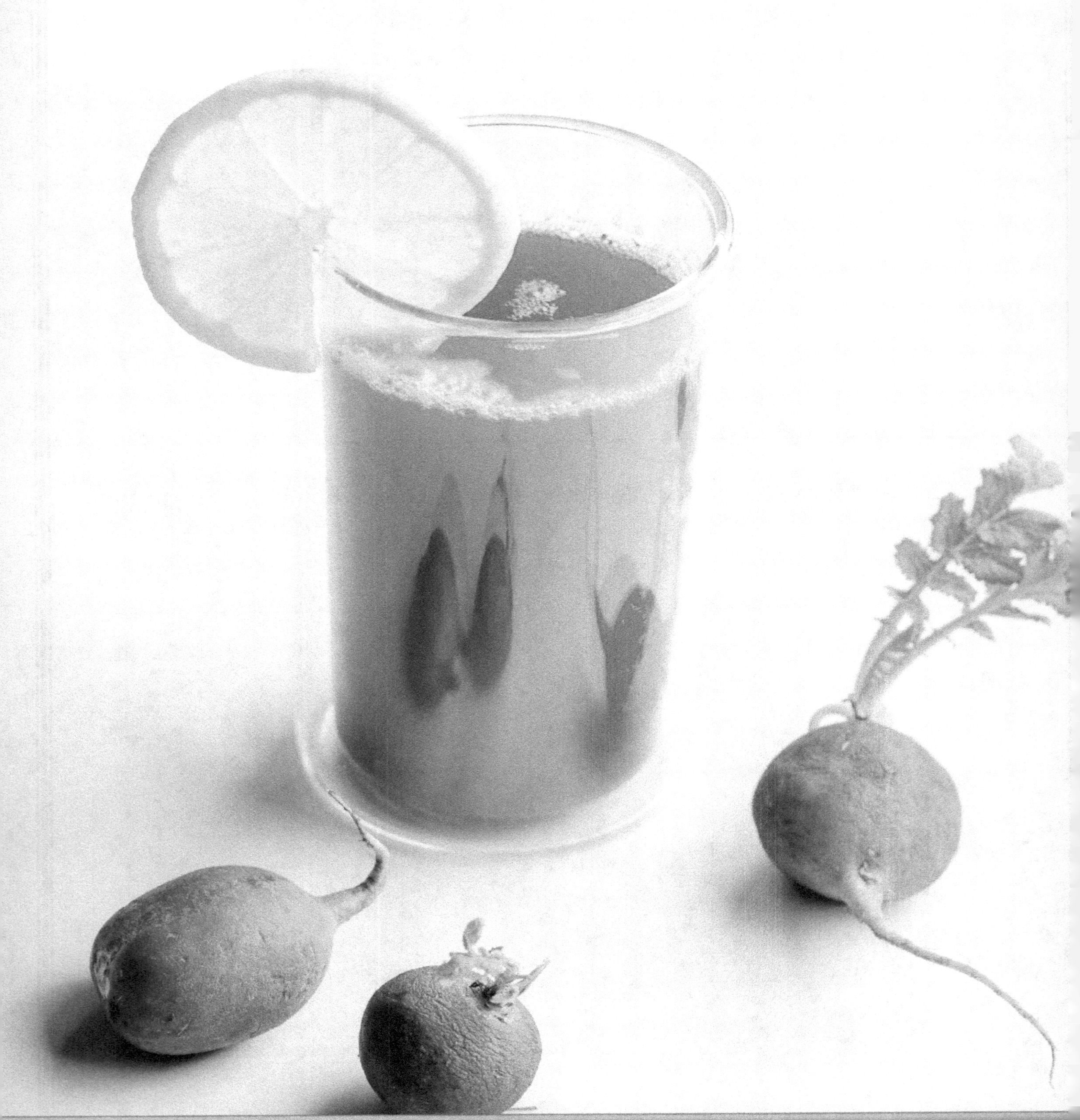
PAULA J. EVANS

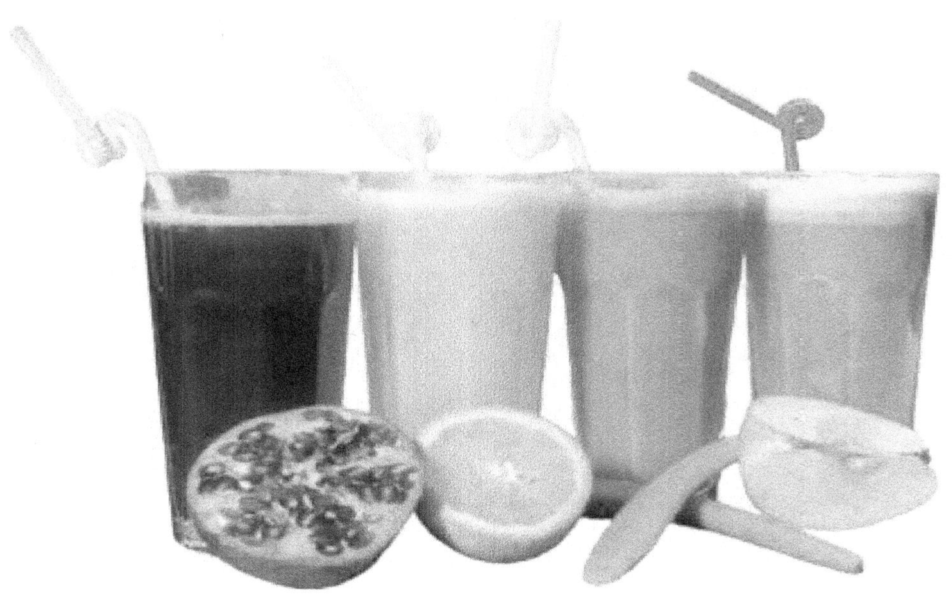

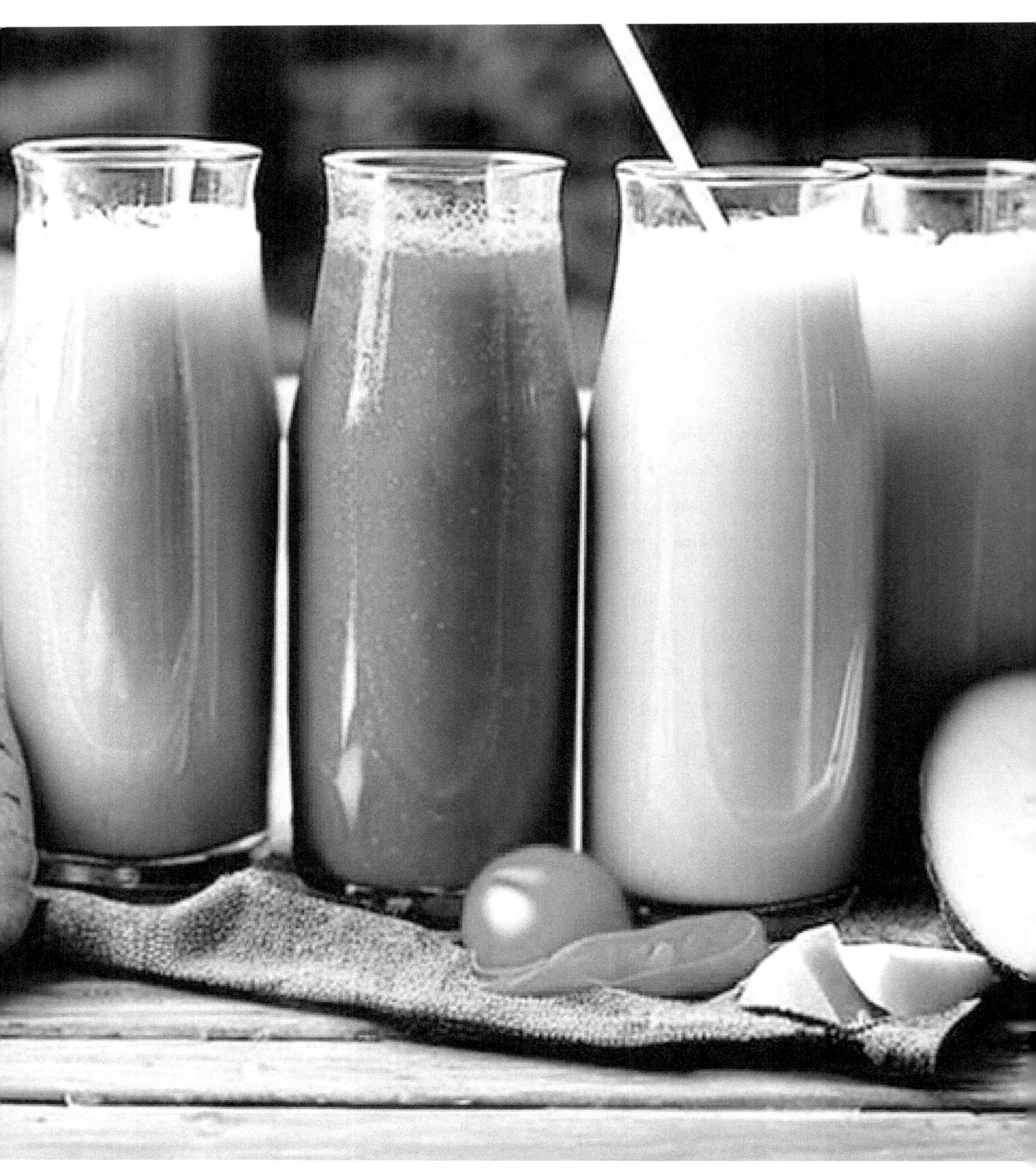

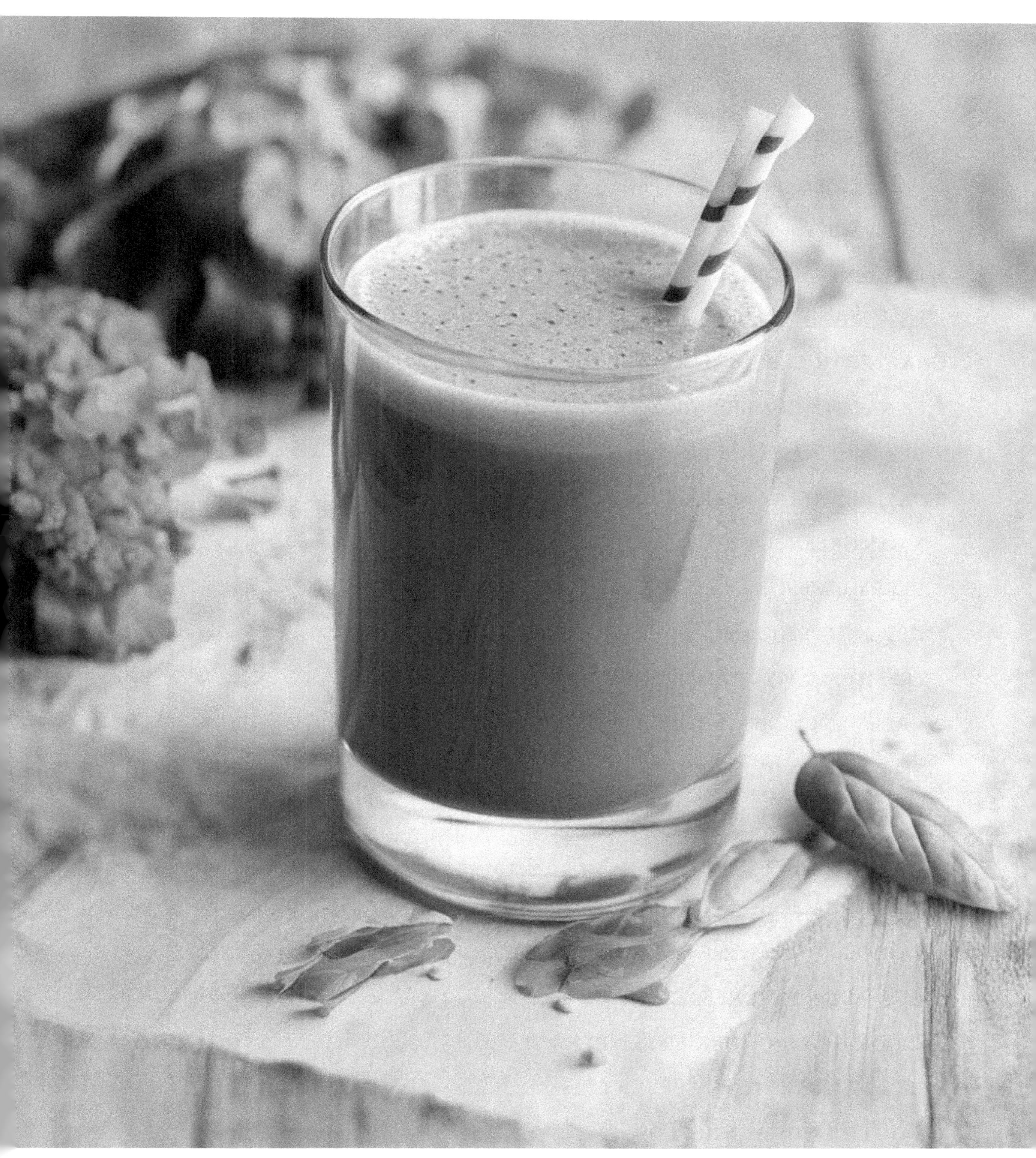

TABLE OF CONTENTS

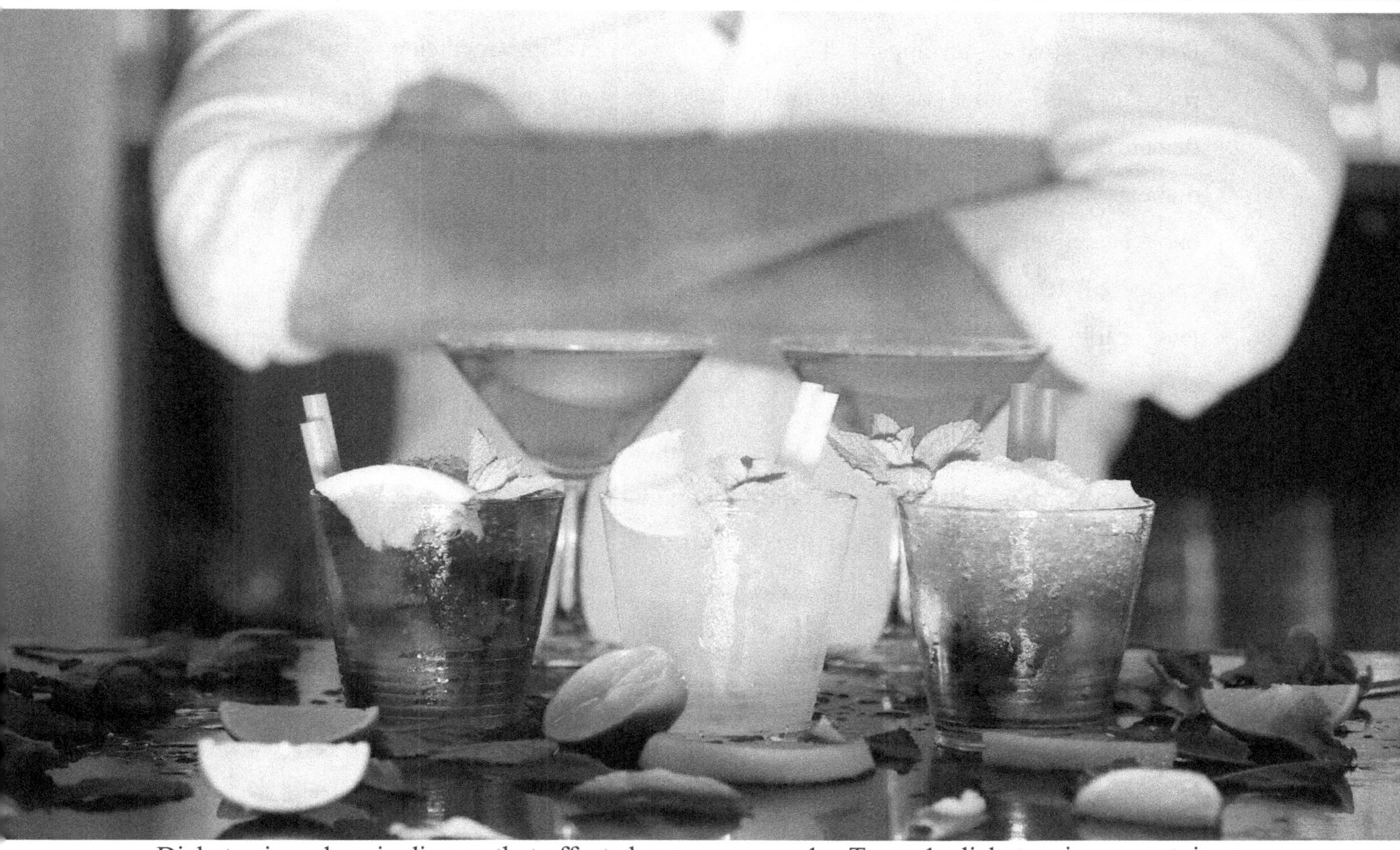

Diabetes is a chronic disease that affects how your body converts food into energy. The majority of the food you consume is converted into glucose, or sugar, and then released into your circulation. When your blood sugar levels rise, your pancreas produces insulin. Insulin functions as a key to unlock the door to your body's cells, allowing glucose to enter and be utilized for energy.

Diabetes Types

Diabetes is classified into three types:

1. Type 1 diabetes is an autoimmune illness in which the body's immune system assaults and kills insulin-producing pancreatic cells. People with type 1 diabetes must take insulin every day to keep their blood sugar levels under control.

2. Type 2 diabetes: The most prevalent kind of diabetes, characterized by a combination of insulin resistance and deficiency. Insulin resistance occurs when the cells of the body do not react

effectively to insulin. Insulin deficit occurs when the body fails to create enough insulin.

3. Diabetes that develops during pregnancy is known as gestational diabetes. Although gestational diabetes normally disappears once the baby is delivered, it might raise the chance of acquiring type 2 diabetes later in life.

Weight Loss

Diabetes patients, particularly those with type 2 diabetes, must lose weight. Even a little amount of weight reduction may improve blood sugar management, lower the risk of complications, and make the disease simpler to manage.

There are several approaches to losing weight, but the ideal strategy is to discover a healthy and sustainable plan that you can keep to in the long run.

Some weight loss strategies for diabetics include:

- Consume complete, unprocessed foods such as fruits, vegetables, whole grains, and lean protein to maintain a healthy diet. Limit your intake of processed meals, fizzy drinks, and harmful fats.

- Regular exercise: On most days of the week, aim for at least 30 minutes of moderate-intensity exercise.

- Taking medicine: Your doctor may prescribe medication if you need assistance regulating your blood sugar levels.

Importance of Juicing

Juicing may be a healthy method to eat fruits and vegetables, but it is vital for diabetics to pick the correct components and quantity amounts.

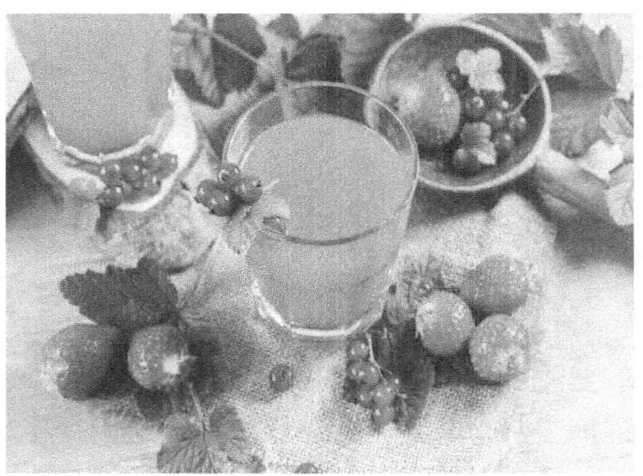

Fruit juice is heavy in sugar and carbs, so restrict your consumption. Mixing fruit juice with water or unsweetened vegetable juice is one method. Berries are a good example of a fruit that is low in sugar.

Vegetable juice is a wonderful choice for diabetics since it is low in sugar and carbs while being rich in nutrients. Carrots, celery, spinach, kale, and cucumber are all excellent juicing veggies.

If you're thinking about juicing, go to your doctor first to make sure it's safe for you and to receive tips on how to pick the correct components and amount proportions.

- Choose fruits and vegetables that are low in sugar.
- Fruit juice should be mixed with water or unsweetened vegetable juice.
- Fruit juice should be consumed in moderation.
- Vegetable juice should be consumed in moderation.
- Before you begin juicing, consult with your doctor.

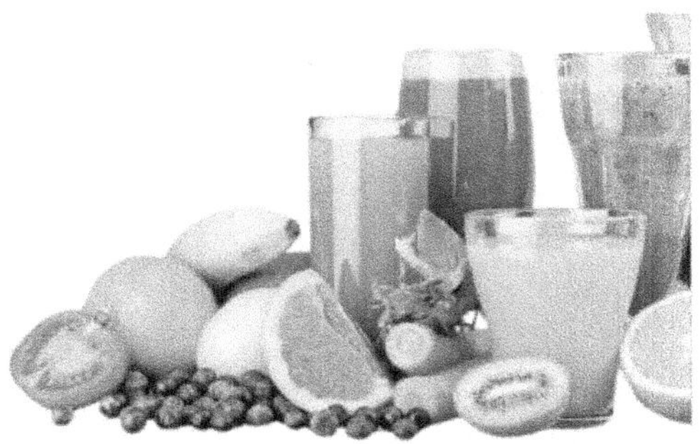

Diabetes is a chronic medical illness that may have serious consequences in a person's life. People with diabetes, with adequate care, may live long and healthy lives. Juicing may be a healthy method to eat fruits and vegetables while also losing weight, which is an essential element of diabetes management. If you're thinking about juicing, see your doctor first to learn how to pick the correct components and quantity quantities.

1. Simple Absorption - Because juices lack fiber, they are readily absorbed by the body. They bypass digestion and enter the cells in less than 30 minutes. The digestion process is interrupted, providing your body additional energy for cleaning, detoxification, and physical exercise.
2. Improved Nutrient Absorption - Juices are beneficial if your digestive system is weak. When you have illnesses like ulcers, reflux, and others, the nutrients in your meal pass out. Juices help you absorb nutrients.
3. alkalinity - Juicing creates an alkaline environment in the body, which improves the immune system and increases energy while decreasing inflammation and discomfort.

four. hydration Juicing hydrates your cells, which improves cell function. Your body need water, which is provided by fresh fruit and vegetable juice. At the same time, juices deliver minerals, vitamins, phytochemicals, and enzymes that your body need.

4. Micronutrients Cooking and preparing food affects micronutrients, making it more difficult for the body to absorb them. Juicing preserves micronutrients.

5. Detoxification - Juicing is an efficient detoxification method. It cleanses the colon and digestive system, boosting the body's metabolism.

6. Chlorophyll - Chlorophyll is a unique structure found in plants. It increases the body's capacity to produce hemoglobin, hence improving oxygen supply to the cells. This provides greater energy to the body.

7. Antioxidants (viii) Antioxidants found in fruits and vegetables help to combat dangerous free radicals. This decreases cell damage, which delays aging or cancer susceptibility.

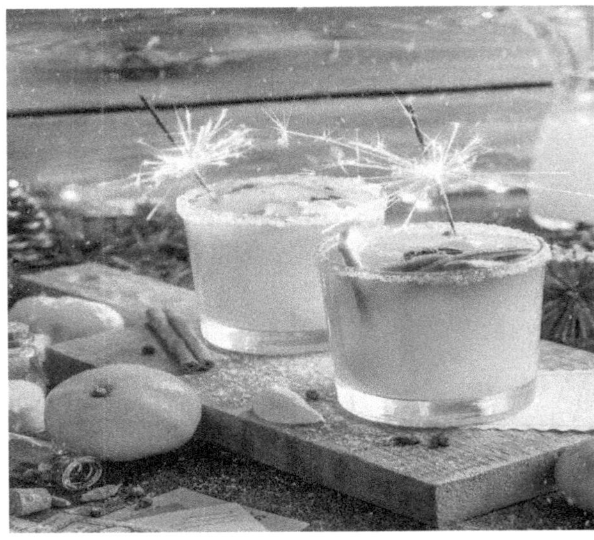

8. Healing effects - Fruits and vegetables have anti-inflammatory effects.

9. Juicing allows you to make a personalized prescription for a certain bodily requirement. This boosts immunity while also strengthening bones and increasing vitality. When you can blend meals, your body can absorb nutrients that aid in healing.

10. Volume - You may devour enormous amounts of veggies and fruits that you would not normally eat. Your body receives nutrients that are necessary for optimal health. The enzymes, minerals, and vitamins found in juices are abundant. Because these nutrients reach your circulation fast, your body reaps the advantages right away.

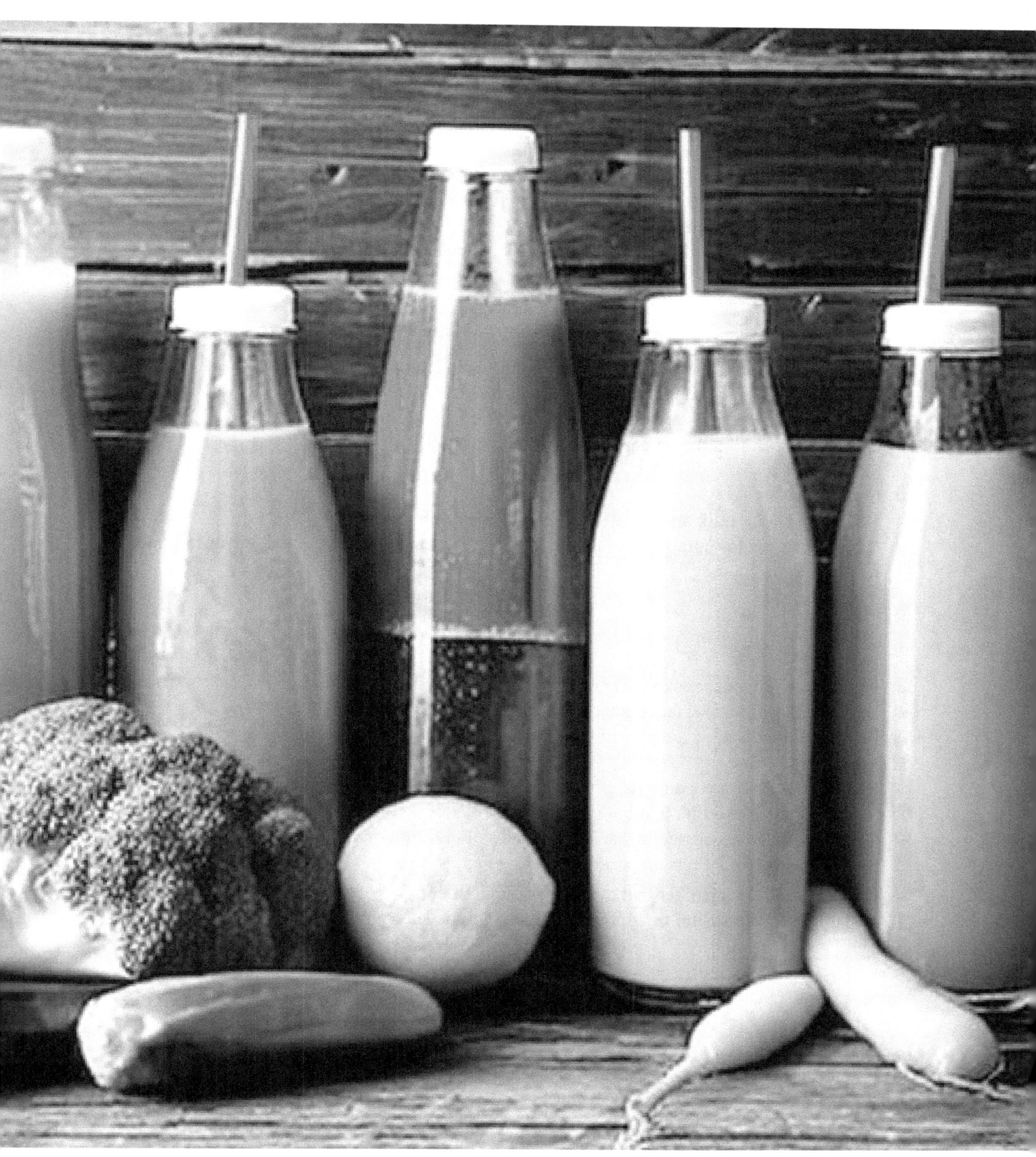

Foods to Avoid, Eat, and Consume in Moderation:

Foods to avoid include:

- Rice, white bread, and spaghetti
- Sugary beverages including soda, juice, and sports drinks
- Candy, chips, and cookies are examples of processed foods.
- Fried meats and vegetables, such as chicken nuggets and French fries
- Cream cheese and butter are examples of full-fat dairy products.
- Butter, lard, coconut oil, and processed foods include saturated and harmful fats.

Foods to consume:

- Brown rice, quinoa, and oats are examples of whole grains.
- Berries, apples, and oranges are examples of fruits.
- Broccoli, spinach, and carrots are examples of vegetables.
- Chicken, fish, and turkey are examples of lean meats.
- Seeds and nuts
- Eggs
- Yogurt and skim milk are examples of low-fat dairy products.
- Olive oil, avocados, almonds, and seeds are high in monounsaturated and polyunsaturated fats.

Foods to consume in moderation:

- Potatoes and maize are examples of starchy veggies.
- Dairy items with a low fat content, such as cheese and yogurt
- Beans and lentils are examples of legumes.
- Meat that is red
- Cream and butter are examples of high-fat dairy products.
- Saturated fats like butter and lard
- Coconut oil and processed meals are examples of unhealthy fats.
- Sugary meals like sweets and cake
- It is essential to remember that everyone's requirements vary, and it is recommended to consult with your doctor or a qualified dietitian to develop a meal plan that is ideal for you.

SPINACH CUCUMBER JUICE

- Preparation Time: 5 minutes
- Serving Size: 1
- Cooking Time: 0 minutes

INGREDIENTS:

- 2 cups fresh spinach leaves
- 1 cucumber, peeled and chopped
- 1 cup water

NUTRITIONAL VALUES (PER SERVING):

- Calories: 40
- Carbohydrates: 8g
- Fiber: 3g
- Protein: 2g
- Fat: 0.5g

INSTRUCTIONS:

1. Wash Spinach: Wash spinach leaves thoroughly.
2. Chop Cucumber: Peel and chop the cucumber.
3. Blend: In a blender, combine spinach, cucumber, and water.
4. Blend Until Smooth: Blend until smooth.
5. Strain (Optional): Strain and serve over ice.

BERRY SPINACH JUICE

- Preparation Time: 7 minutes
- Serving Size: 1
- Cooking Time: 0 minutes

INGREDIENTS:

- 1 cup mixed berries (strawberries, blueberries, raspberries)
- 1 cup fresh spinach leaves
- 1/2 cup water

NUTRITIONAL VALUES (PER SERVING):

- Calories: 60
- Carbohydrates: 14g
- Fiber: 4g
- Protein: 2g
- Fat: 0.5g

INSTRUCTIONS:

1. Rinse Berries and Spinach: Rinse berries and spinach leaves.
2. Blend: In a blender, combine berries, spinach, and water.
3. Blend Until Smooth: Blend until smooth.
4. Strain (Optional): Strain and enjoy.

PARSLEY STRAWBERRIES PINEAPPLE JUICE

- Preparation Time: 8 minutes
- Serving Size: 1
- Cooking Time: 0 minutes

INGREDIENTS:

- 1 cup fresh parsley leaves
- 1 cup strawberries, hulled
- 1 cup fresh pineapple, chopped 1/2 cup water

NUTRITIONAL VALUES (PER SERVING):

- Calories: 50
- Carbohydrates: 12g
- Fiber: 3g
- Protein: 1g
- Fat: 0.5g

INSTRUCTIONS:

1. Wash parsley, hull strawberries, and chop pineapple.
2. Blend: In a blender, combine parsley, strawberries, pineapple, and water.
3. Blend Until Smooth: Blend until a smooth consistency is achieved.
4. Strain (Optional): Strain the juice for a smoother texture.
5. Serve: Pour into a glass and enjoy.

MEAN GREEN JUICE

- Preparation Time: 10 minutes
- Serving Size: 1
- Cooking Time: 0 minutes

INGREDIENTS:

- 1 cup kale leaves
- 2 celery stalks
- 1 cucumber, peeled
- 1/2 lemon, peeled
- 1 cup water

NUTRITIONAL VALUES (PER SERVING):

- Calories: 45
- Carbohydrates: 10g
- Fiber: 4g
- Protein: 2g
- Fat: 0.5g

INSTRUCTIONS:

1. Wash and Chop: Wash kale, celery, and cucumber. Peel lemon.
2. Prepare Ingredients: Chop vegetables into smaller pieces.
3. Blend: In a blender, combine kale, celery, cucumber, lemon, and water.
4. Blend Until Smooth: Blend until a smooth consistency is achieved.

5. Strain (Optional): Strain the juice for a smoother texture.

6. Serve: Pour into a glass and enjoy.

BERRY LIME JUICE

- Preparation Time: 6 minutes
- Serving Size: 1
- Cooking Time: 0 minutes

INGREDIENTS:

- 1 cup mixed berries (blueberries, raspberries)
- 1 lime, juiced
- 1/2 cup water

NUTRITIONAL VALUES (PER SERVING):

- Calories: 45
- Carbohydrates: 11g
- Fiber: 3g
- Protein: 1g
- Fat: 0.5g

INSTRUCTIONS:

1. Rinse Berries: Rinse mixed berries thoroughly.

2. Juice Lime: Extract juice from the lime.

3. Blend: In a blender, combine berries, lime juice, and water.

4. Blend Until Smooth: Blend until a smooth consistency is achieved.

5. Strain (Optional): Strain the juice for a smoother texture.

6. Serve: Pour into a glass and enjoy.

GREEN APPLE JUICE

- Preparation Time: 5 minutes
- Serving Size: 1
- Cooking Time: 0 minutes

INGREDIENTS:

- 2 green apples, cored 1/2 lemon, peeled 1 cup water

NUTRITIONAL VALUES (PER SERVING):

- Calories: 60
- Carbohydrates: 15g
- Fiber: 3g
- Protein: 1g
- Fat: 0.5g

INSTRUCTIONS:

1. Core Apples: Core green apples.

2. Peel Lemon: Peel the lemon.

3. Blend: In a blender, combine green apples, lemon, and water.
4. Blend Until Smooth: Blend until a smooth consistency is achieved.
5. Strain (Optional): Strain the juice for a smoother texture.
6. Serve: Pour into a glass and enjoy.

FRESH CREAMY CARROT JUICE

- Preparation Time: 7 minutes
- Serving Size: 1
- Cooking Time: 0 minutes

INGREDIENTS:

- 3 large carrots, peeled and chopped
- 1/2 cup unsweetened almond milk
- 1/2 teaspoon cinnamon (optional)

NUTRITIONAL VALUES (PER SERVING):

- Calories: 70
- Carbohydrates: 16g
- Fiber: 4g
- Protein: 2g
- Fat: 1g

INSTRUCTIONS:

1. Prepare Carrots: Peel and chop carrots.
2. Blend: In a blender, combine chopped carrots, almond milk, and cinnamon.
3. Blend Until Smooth: Blend until a creamy consistency is achieved.
4. Strain (Optional): Strain for a smoother texture.
5. Serve: Pour into a glass and enjoy the creamy goodness.

GREEN STRING BEANS JUICE

- Preparation Time: 8 minutes
- Serving Size: 1
- Cooking Time: 0 minutes

INGREDIENTS:

- 1 cup green string beans, ends trimmed
- 1/2 cucumber, peeled 1/2 lime, juiced
- 1/2 cup water

NUTRITIONAL VALUES (PER SERVING):

- Calories: 40
- Carbohydrates: 9g
- Fiber: 3g
- Protein: 2g

1. Trim String Beans: Trim the ends of green string beans.
2. Prepare Cucumber: Peel and chop cucumber.
3. Juice Lime: Extract juice from the lime.
4. Blend: In a blender, combine string beans, cucumber, lime juice, and water.
5. Blend Until Smooth: Blend until a smooth consistency is achieved.
6. Strain (Optional): Strain the juice for a smoother texture.
7. Serve: Pour into a glass and enjoy the unique blend.

SPICED TOMATO JUICE

- Preparation Time: 5 minutes
- Serving Size: 1
- Cooking Time: 0 minutes

INGREDIENTS:

- 2 large tomatoes, chopped
- 1/2 teaspoon cayenne pepper
- 1/2 teaspoon black pepper
- 1/2 teaspoon sea salt
- 1/2 cup water

NUTRITIONAL VALUES (PER SERVING):

- Calories: 35
- Carbohydrates: 8g
- Fiber: 2g
- Protein: 1g
- Fat: 0.5g

INSTRUCTIONS:

1. Chop Tomatoes: Chop tomatoes into smaller pieces.
2. Spice It Up: Add cayenne pepper, black pepper, and sea salt.
3. Blend: In a blender, combine chopped tomatoes, spices, and water.
4. Blend Until Smooth: Blend until a smooth consistency is achieved.
5. Strain (Optional): Strain for a smoother texture.
6. Serve: Pour into a glass and savor the spiced tomato goodness.

WATERMELON JUICE

- Preparation Time: 5 minutes

INGREDIENTS:

- 2 cups fresh watermelon, diced
- 1/2 lime, juiced Mint leaves for garnish (optional)

NUTRITIONAL VALUES (PER SERVING):

- Calories: 50
- Carbohydrates: 12g
- Fiber: 1g
- Protein: 1g
- Fat: 0.5g

INSTRUCTIONS:

1. Dice Watermelon: Dice fresh watermelon into cubes.
2. Juice Lime: Extract juice from the lime.
3. Blend: In a blender, combine diced watermelon and lime juice.
4. Blend Until Smooth: Blend until a smooth consistency is achieved.
5. Strain (Optional): Strain for a smoother texture.
6. Garnish (Optional): Add mint leaves for a refreshing touch.
7. Serve: Pour into a glass and enjoy the hydrating watermelon delight.

CITRUS BEET BLAST JUICE

⚬ Preparation Time: 8 minutes

⚬ Serving Size: 1

⚬ Cooking Time: 0 minutes

INGREDIENTS:

- 1 medium-sized beet, peeled and chopped
- 1 orange, peeled and segmented
- 1/2 lemon, peeled 1/2-inch ginger, peeled 1 cup water

NUTRITIONAL VALUES (PER SERVING):

- Calories: 70
- Carbohydrates: 18g
- Fiber: 4g
- Protein: 2g
- Fat: 0.5g

INSTRUCTIONS:

1. Prepare Beet: Peel and chop the beet.
2. Prepare Citrus: Peel and segment the orange. Peel the lemon.
3. Chop Ginger: Peel and chop the ginger.
4. Blend: In a blender, combine chopped beet, orange segments, lemon, ginger, and water.

5. Blend Until Smooth: Blend until a smooth consistency is achieved.

6. Strain (Optional): Strain for a smoother texture.

7. Serve: Pour into a glass and enjoy the vibrant citrus beet blend.

MANGO BASIL BLISS JUICE

INGREDIENTS:

- 1 cup fresh mango, diced
- 1/4 cup fresh basil leaves
- 1/2 lime, juiced 1/2 cup water

NUTRITIONAL VALUES (PER SERVING):

- Calories: 80
- Carbohydrates: 20g
- Fiber: 3g
- Protein: 1g
- Fat: 0.5g

INSTRUCTIONS:

1. Dice Mango: Dice fresh mango into cubes.

2. Prepare Basil: Wash and prepare fresh basil leaves.

3. Juice Lime: Extract juice from the lime.

4. Blend: In a blender, combine diced mango, basil leaves, lime juice, and water.

5. Blend Until Smooth: Blend until a smooth consistency is achieved.

6. Strain (Optional): Strain for a smoother texture.

7. Serve: Pour into a glass and relish the mango basil bliss.

TURMERIC PINEAPPLE PARADISE JUICE

- Preparation Time: 7 minutes
- Serving Size: 1
- Cooking Time: 0 minutes

INGREDIENTS:

- 1 cup fresh pineapple, diced
- 1/2 teaspoon ground turmeric
- 1/2 teaspoon honey (optional)
- 1/2 cup water

NUTRITIONAL VALUES (PER SERVING):

- Calories: 60

- Carbohydrates: 15g
- Fiber: 2g
- Protein: 1g
- Fat: 0.5g

INSTRUCTIONS:

- Dice Pineapple: Dice fresh pineapple into cubes.
- Add Turmeric: Incorporate ground turmeric.
- Optional Sweetener: Add honey if desired.
- Blend: In a blender, combine diced pineapple, turmeric, honey, and water.
- Blend Until Smooth: Blend until a smooth consistency is achieved.
- Strain (Optional): Strain for a smoother texture.
- Serve: Pour into a glass and savor the tropical turmeric delight.

CUCUMBER MINT REFRESHER JUICE

- Preparation Time: 6 minutes
- Serving Size: 1
- Cooking Time: 0 minutes

INGREDIENTS:

- 1 cucumber, peeled and chopped
- 1/4 cup fresh mint leaves
- 1/2 lime, juiced
- 1/2 teaspoon agave nectar (optional)
- 1 cup water

NUTRITIONAL VALUES (PER SERVING):

- Calories: 30
- Carbohydrates: 8g
- Fiber: 2g
- Protein: 1g
- Fat: 0.5g

INSTRUCTIONS:

1. Prepare Cucumber: Peel and chop the cucumber.
2. Prepare Mint: Wash and prepare fresh mint leaves.
3. Juice Lime: Extract juice from the lime.
4. Optional Sweetener: Add agave nectar if desired.
5. Blend: In a blender, combine chopped cucumber, mint leaves, lime juice, agave nectar, and water.
6. Blend Until Smooth: Blend until a smooth consistency is achieved.
7. Strain (Optional): Strain for a smoother texture.
8. Serve: Pour into a glass and enjoy the crisp cucumber mint refresher.

ORANGE CARROT GINGER ELIXIR JUICE

- Preparation Time: 8 minutes
- Serving Size: 1
- Cooking Time: 0 minutes

INGREDIENTS:

- 2 large carrots, peeled and chopped
- 1 orange, peeled and segmented
- 1/2-inch ginger, peeled
- 1/2 teaspoon turmeric powder
- 1 cup water

NUTRITIONAL VALUES (PER SERVING):

- Calories: 65
- Carbohydrates: 15g
- Fiber: 4g
- Protein: 2g
- Fat: 0.5g

INSTRUCTIONS:

1. Prepare Carrots: Peel and chop carrots.
2. Prepare Orange: Peel and segment the orange.
3. Chop Ginger: Peel and chop ginger.
4. Add Turmeric: Incorporate turmeric powder.
5. Blend: In a blender, combine chopped carrots, orange segments, ginger, turmeric, and water.
6. Blend Until Smooth: Blend until a smooth consistency is achieved.
7. Strain (Optional): Strain for a smoother texture.
8. Serve: Pour into a glass and relish the zesty orange carrot elixir.

BLUEBERRY KALE POWER JUICE

- Preparation Time: 7 minutes
- Serving Size: 1
- Cooking Time: 0 minutes

INGREDIENTS:

- 1 cup blueberries
- 1 cup kale leaves
- 1/2 banana
- 1/2 cup water

NUTRITIONAL VALUES (PER SERVING):

- Calories: 70
- Carbohydrates: 17g
- Fiber: 4g
- Protein: 2g
- Fat: 0.5g

1. Rinse Blueberries and Kale: Rinse blueberries and kale leaves thoroughly.
2. Peel Banana: Peel and chop the banana.
3. Blend: In a blender, combine blueberries, kale leaves, banana, and water.
4. Blend Until Smooth: Blend until a smooth consistency is achieved.
5. Strain (Optional): Strain for a smoother texture.
6. Serve: Pour into a glass and experience the nutritious blueberry kale power.

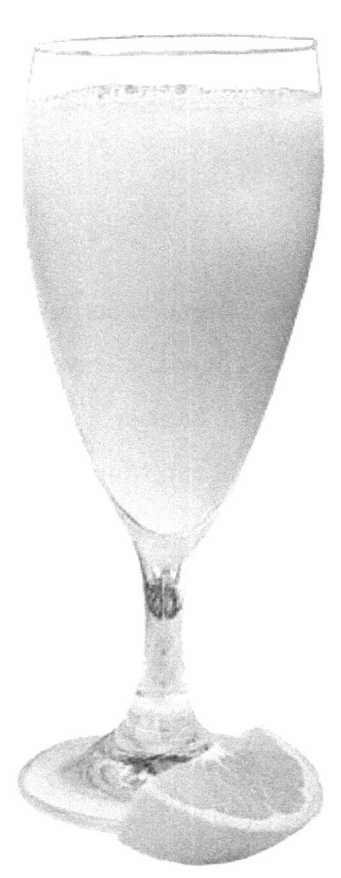
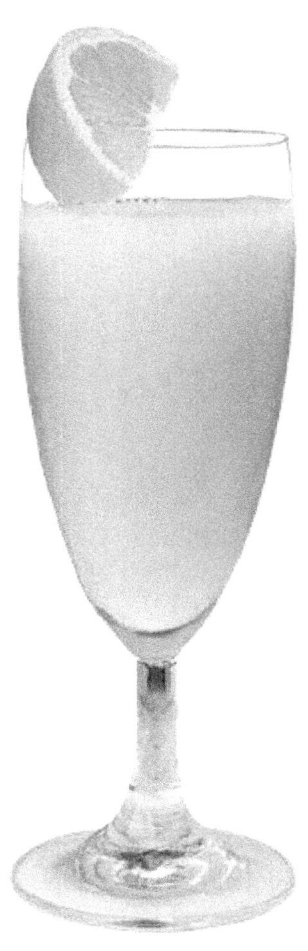

SLIMMING JUICE FROM BEETS AND CARROTS

- Time to Prepare: 10 minutes
- 1 serving size
- Time to cook: 0 minutes

INGREDIENTS:

- 1 medium peeled and chopped beetroot
- 2 medium peeled and sliced carrots
- 1 lemon (peeled)
- 1 inch peeled ginger
- 1 cup of water

NUTRITIONAL INFORMATION (PER SERVING):

- 60 calories
- 14g carbohydrate
- 4g fiber
- 2g protein
- Fat: 0.5g

INSTRUCTIONS:

1. Prepare the vegetables by peeling and chopping the beets and carrots.
2. Lemon and Ginger Preparation: Peel the lemon and ginger.
3. Blend beets, carrots, lemon, ginger, and water in a blender.
4. Blend Until Smooth: Blend until the mixture is smooth.
5. Optional straining: Strain for a smoother texture.
6. Pour this slimming beetroot and carrot combination into a glass and enjoy.

WEIGHT LOSS WITH GARDEN APPLE AND CARROT JUICE

- Time to Prepare: 8 minutes
- 1 serving size
- Time to cook: 0 minutes

INGREDIENTS:

- 1 apple, cored and cut from the garden
- 2 medium peeled and sliced carrots
- 1 lemon (peeled)
- 1 cup of water

NUTRITIONAL INFORMATION (PER SERVING):

- 50 calories
- 12g carbohydrate
- 3g fiber

- 1g protein
- Fat: 0.5g

INSTRUCTIONS:

1. Apple and carrot preparation: Core and cut the apple. Carrots should be peeled and chopped.
2. Lemon Preparation: Peel the lemon.
3. Blend the apple, carrots, lemon, and water in a blender.
4. Blend Until Smooth: Blend until the mixture is smooth.
5. Optional straining: Strain for a smoother texture.
6. Pour into a glass and enjoy this delicious apple and carrot mixture, which is ideal for weight reduction.

JUICE WITH CUCUMBER PROTEIN

- Time to Prepare: 5 minutes
- 1 serving size
- Time to cook: 0 minutes

INGREDIENTS:

- 1 peeled and sliced cucumber
- 1/2 cup plain Greek yogurt
- 1 teaspoon chia seeds
- Optional: 1/2 teaspoon honey
- 1 cup of water

NUTRITIONAL INFORMATION (PER SERVING):

- 80 calories
- 10g carbohydrate
- 4g fiber
- 6g protein
- Fat: 3.5g

INSTRUCTIONS:

1. Cucumber Preparation: Peel and cut the cucumber.
2. Add Greek yogurt and chia seeds for a protein boost.
3. Optional Sweetener: If desired, add honey.
4. Blend cucumber, Greek yogurt, chia seeds, honey, and water in a blender.
5. Blend Until Smooth: Blend until the mixture is smooth.
6. Pour into a glass and enjoy this protein-packed cucumber juice, which is perfect for weight reduction with additional protein.

SLIMMING JUICE MADE WITH APPLES AND CUCUMBERS

- Time to Prepare: 6 minutes
- 1 serving size
- Time to cook: 0 minutes

INGREDIENTS:

- 1 cored and chopped apple
- 1/2 peeled and sliced cucumber
- 1 lime (juiced)
- 1 tablespoon flaxseeds
- 1 cup of water

NUTRITIONAL INFORMATION (PER SERVING):

- 70 calories
- 18g carbohydrate
- 4g fiber
- 1g protein
- Fat: 0.5g

INSTRUCTIONS:

1. Apple and cucumber preparation: Core and cut the apple. Peel and finely slice the cucumber.
2. Lime Juice: Extract the juice from the lime.
3. Flaxseeds: Include flaxseeds for extra fiber.
4. Blend the apple, cucumber, lime juice, flaxseeds, and water in a blender.
5. Blend Until Smooth: Blend until the mixture is smooth.
6. Pour into a glass and enjoy this apples and cucumber combination, which is ideal for individuals looking to lose weight.

PINEAPPLE REFRESHER JUICE FOR WEIGHT LOSS

- Time to Prepare: 7 minutes
- 1 serving size
- Time to cook: 0 minutes

INGREDIENTS:

- 1 cup diced fresh pineapple
- 1 tablespoon cayenne pepper
- 14 cup apple cider vinegar
- Optional: 1/2 teaspoon honey
- 1 cup of water

NUTRITIONAL INFORMATION (PER SERVING):

- 50 calories
- 13g carbohydrate
- 2g fiber

- 1g protein
- Fat: 0.5g

INSTRUCTIONS:

1. Pineapple Dice: Cut fresh pineapple into cubes.
2. Add cayenne pepper to kick start your metabolism.
3. Apple Cider Vinegar: Include apple cider vinegar in your diet for its possible weight reduction advantages.
4. Optional Sweetener: If desired, add honey.
5. Blend the chopped pineapple, cayenne pepper, apple cider vinegar, honey, and water in a blender.
6. Blend Until Smooth: Blend until the mixture is smooth.
7. Pour into a glass and enjoy this tropical-inspired weight loss refreshment.

WEIGHT LOSS JUICE WITH VEGETABLE FUSION

- Time to Prepare: 8 minutes
- 1 serving size
- Time to cook: 0 minutes

INGREDIENTS:

- 1 medium-sized chopped tomato
- 1/2 peeled and sliced cucumber
- 1/2 chopped bell pepper, any color
- 1/2 peeled and sliced carrot
- 1 lemon (peeled)
- 1 cup of water

NUTRITIONAL INFORMATION (PER SERVING):

- 40 calories
- 9g Carbohydrates
- 3g fiber
- 2g protein
- Fat: 0.5g

INSTRUCTIONS:

1. Chop the following vegetables: tomato, cucumber, bell pepper, carrot, and lemon.
2. Blend chopped veggies and water in a blender.
3. Blend Until Smooth: Blend until the mixture is smooth.
4. Optional straining: Strain for a smoother texture.
5. Pour into a glass and enjoy this nutrient-rich vegetable fusion juice as part of your weight reduction strategy.

WATERMELON WEIGHT LOSS JUICE HYDRATING

- Time to Prepare: 5 minutes
- 1 serving size
- Time to cook: 0 minutes

INGREDIENTS:

- 2 cups sliced fresh watermelon
- 1/2 peeled and sliced cucumber
- 1 lime (juiced)
- 1 tablespoon fresh mint
- 1 cup of water

NUTRITIONAL INFORMATION (PER SERVING):

- 45 calories
- 11g carbohydrate
- 1g fiber
- 1g protein
- Fat: 0.5g

INSTRUCTIONS:

1. Watermelon Dice: Cut fresh watermelon into cubes.
2. Cucumber Preparation: Peel and cut the cucumber.
3. Lime Juice: Extract the juice from the lime.
4. Mint Leaves: For a refreshing taste, add mint leaves.
5. Blend: Combine diced watermelon, cucumber, lime juice, mint leaves, and water in a blender.
6. Blend Until Smooth: Blend until the mixture is smooth.
7. Pour into a glass and enjoy the moisturizing watermelon treat, ideal for assisting you on your weight reduction path.

FAT-BURNING GRAPEFRUIT JUICE

- Time to Prepare: 6 minutes
- 1 serving size
- Time to cook: 0 minutes

INGREDIENTS:

- 1 peeled and segmented pink grapefruit
- 1/2 peeled and sliced cucumber
- Optional: 1/2 teaspoon honey
- 1 cup of water

NUTRITIONAL INFORMATION (PER SERVING):

- 60 calories
- 15g carbohydrate
- 3g fiber
- 1g protein

INSTRUCTIONS:

1. Grapefruit Preparation: Peel and slice the pink grapefruit.
2. Cucumber Preparation: Peel and cut the cucumber.
3. Optional Sweetener: If desired, add honey.
4. Blend grapefruit segments, cucumber, honey, and water in a blender.
5. Blend Until Smooth: Blend until the mixture is smooth.
6. Pour this fat-burning grapefruit juice into a glass and enjoy as a delightful complement to your weight reduction program.

SLIMMING JUICE FROM KIWI

⚘ Time to Prepare: 7 minutes
⚘ 1 serving size
⚘ Time to cook: 0 minutes

INGREDIENTS:

⚘ 2 peeled and sliced kiwis
⚘ 1/2 peeled and sliced cucumber
⚘ 1 lime (juiced)
⚘ 1 teaspoon chia seeds
⚘ 1 cup of water

NUTRITIONAL INFORMATION (PER SERVING):

⚘ 70 calories
⚘ 16g carbohydrate
⚘ 5g fiber
⚘ 2g protein
⚘ Fat: 1g

INSTRUCTIONS:

1. Prepare the kiwis by peeling and slicing them.
2. Cucumber Preparation: Peel and cut the cucumber.
3. Lime Juice: Extract the juice from the lime.
4. Include Chia Seeds: Chia seeds provide fiber and texture.
5. Blend sliced kiwis, diced cucumber, lime juice, chia seeds, and water in a blender.
6. Blend Until Smooth: Blend until the mixture is smooth.
7. Pour into a glass and enjoy this kiwi slimming juice, a healthy and delightful option for weight reduction.

METABOLISM BOOSTER JUICE WITH MINT

INGREDIENTS:

- 1 cup berries (strawberries and blueberries)
- 1 apple, cored and diced
- 1/2 peeled and sliced cucumber
- 1 tablespoon mint leaves, fresh
- 1 lemon (peeled)
- 1 cup of water

NUTRITIONAL INFORMATION (PER SERVING):

- 55 calories
- 14g carbohydrate
- 3g fiber
- 1g protein
- Fat: 0.5g

INSTRUCTIONS:

1. Rinse Berries: Thoroughly rinse the mixed berries.
2. Apple and cucumber preparation: Core and cut the apple. Peel and finely slice the cucumber.
3. Mint Preparation: Wash and dry fresh mint leaves.
4. Lemon Preparation: Peel the lemon.
5. Blend washed berries, diced apple, chopped cucumber, mint leaves, lemon juice, and water in a blender.
6. Blend Until Smooth: Blend until the mixture is smooth.
7. Pour this metabolism-boosting minty fruit juice into a glass and enjoy.

SLIM-DOWN CITRUS CELERY JUICE

INGREDIENTS:

- 2 peeled and segmented oranges
- 1/2 peeled and sliced grapefruit
- 2 chopped celery stalks
- 1/2 peeled cucumber
- 1 cup of water

NUTRITIONAL INFORMATION (PER SERVING):

- 70 calories
- 18g carbohydrate
- 4g fiber

- 2g protein
- Fat: 0.5g

INSTRUCTIONS:

- Peel and segment oranges and grapefruit for preparation.
- Celery stalks should be chopped.
- Cucumber Preparation: Peel and cut cucumber.
- Blend: Combine segments oranges and grapefruit, diced celery, peeled cucumber, and water in a blender.
- Blend Until Smooth: Blend until the mixture is smooth.
- Optional: Strain the juice to get a smoother texture.
- Pour into a glass and enjoy this citrus celery slim-down juice, a tasty solution for individuals seeking to lose weight.

SLIMMING ELIXIR WITH BERRIES AND SPINACH

- Time to Prepare: 7 minutes
- 1 serving size
- Time to cook: 0 minutes

INGREDIENTS:

- 1 cup berries (strawberries and blueberries)
- a few fresh spinach leaves
- 1 apple, cored and diced
- 1 lime (juiced)
- 1 cup of water

NUTRITIONAL INFORMATION (PER SERVING):

- 55 calories
- 14g carbohydrate
- 3g fiber
- 1g protein
- Fat: 0.5g

INSTRUCTIONS:

1. Rinse Berries: Thoroughly rinse the mixed berries.
2. Wash fresh spinach leaves before preparing them.
3. Prepare the apple by core and chopping it.
4. Lime Juice: Extract the juice from the lime.
5. Blend washed berries, fresh spinach leaves, sliced apple, lime juice, and water in a blender.
6. Blend Until Smooth: Blend until the mixture is smooth.

7. Pour this berry spinach slimming elixir into a glass and enjoy.

FUSION OF TURMERIC AND MANGO

- Time to Prepare: 6 minutes
- 1 serving size
- Time to cook: 0 minutes

INGREDIENTS:

- 1 cup chopped fresh mango
- 1 teaspoon turmeric powder
- a half teaspoon cinnamon
- Optional: 1/2 teaspoon honey
- 1 cup of water

NUTRITIONAL INFORMATION (PER SERVING):

- 80 calories
- 20g carbohydrates
- 3g fiber
- 1g protein
- Fat: 0.5g

INSTRUCTIONS:

1. Mango Dice: Cut fresh mango into cubes.
2. Turmeric and Cinnamon: Mix in ground turmeric and cinnamon.
3. Optional Sweetener: If desired, add honey.
4. Blend the diced mango, ground turmeric, cinnamon, honey, and water in a blender.
5. Blend Until Smooth: Blend until the mixture is smooth.
6. Pour into a glass and enjoy the delectable mix of turmeric and mango.

INFUSION WITH GREEN TEA AND BERRIES

- Time to Prepare: 5 minutes
- 1 serving size
- Time to cook: 0 minutes

INGREDIENTS:

- 1 brewed and cooled green tea bag
- 1 cup berries (strawberries and raspberries)
- 1 lemon (juiced)
- Optional: 1/2 teaspoon honey
- Ice cubes are optional.

NUTRITIONAL INFORMATION (PER SERVING):

- 20 calories
- 5g carbohydrate
- 2g fiber

- 1g protein
- Fat: 0.5g

1. Green Tea: Brew a green tea bag and set it aside to cool.
2. Prepare Berries: Thoroughly rinse the mixed berries.
3. Lemon Juice: Extract the juice from the lemon.
4. Optional Sweetener: If desired, add honey.
5. In a glass, blend the brewed green tea, mixed berries, lemon juice, and honey.
6. Stir well: fully mix.
7. Serve with Ice (Optional): If desired, add ice cubes.
8. Sip this pleasant green tea berry infusion, which is ideal for a light and healthful beverage.

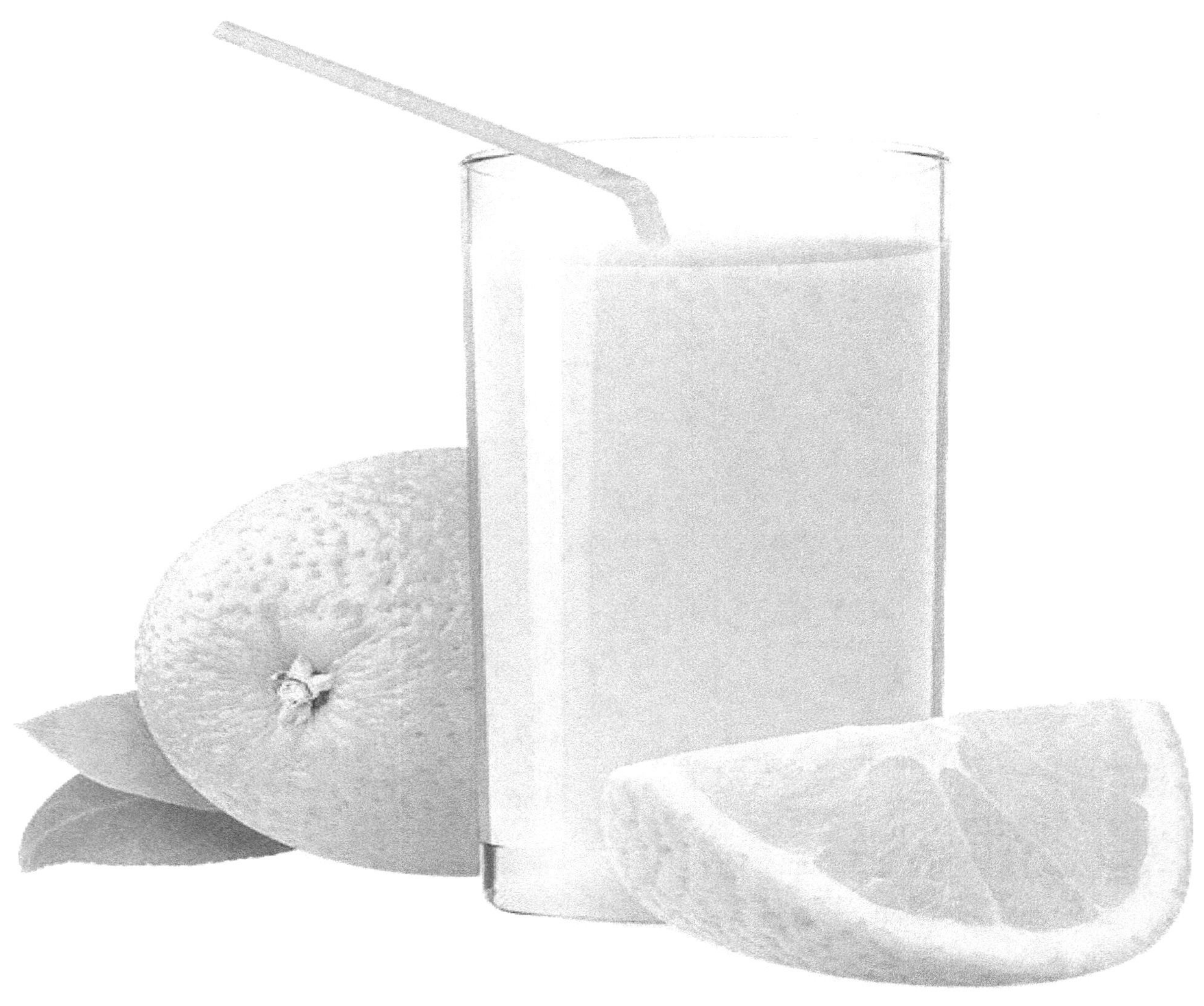

DETOX JUICE WITH CITRUS

- Time to Prepare: 8 minutes
- 1 serving size
- Time to cook: 0 minutes

INGREDIENTS:

- 2 peeled and segmented oranges
- 1 peeled and segmented grapefruit
- 1 lemon (peeled)
- 1 inch peeled ginger
- 1 cup of water

NUTRITIONAL INFORMATION (PER SERVING):

- 70 calories
- 18g carbohydrate
- 4g fiber
- 2g protein
- Fat: 0.5g

INSTRUCTIONS:

1. Peel and segment oranges and grapefruit for preparation.
2. Peel the lemon and ginger and chop them.
3. Blend: Combine segments oranges and grapefruit, peeled lemon, peeled ginger, and water in a blender.
4. Blend Until Smooth: Blend until the mixture is smooth.
5. Optional: Strain the juice to get a smoother texture.
6. Pour this citrus cleanser detox juice into a glass and enjoy.

GREEN GODDESS CLEANSING ELIXIR

- Time to Prepare: 6 minutes
- 1 serving size
- Time to cook: 0 minutes

INGREDIENTS:

- 1 cup fresh kale leaves
- 1/2 peeled and sliced cucumber
- 1 green apple, cored and diced
- 1 lemon (peeled)
- 1 cup of water

NUTRITIONAL INFORMATION (PER SERVING):

- 50 calories
- 12g carbohydrate
- 3g fiber
- 2g protein
- Fat: 0.5g

1. INSTRUCTIONS:

2. Rinse Kale: Thoroughly rinse the kale leaves.

3. Cucumber, Apple, and Lemon Preparation: Peel and cut cucumber. Remove the core and cut the green apple. Lemon should be peeled.

4. In a blender, add the kale leaves, cucumber, green apple, peeled lemon, and water.

5. Blend Until Smooth: Blend until the mixture is smooth.

6. Optional: Strain the juice to get a smoother texture.

7. Pour this green goddess detox elixir into a glass and enjoy.

BLEND OF DETOXIFYING BEETS AND BERRIES

- Time to Prepare: 7 minutes
- 1 serving size
- Time to cook: 0 minutes

INGREDIENTS:

- 1 medium-sized peeled and sliced beet
- 1 cup berries (strawberries, blueberries, and raspberries)
- 1/2 peeled and sliced cucumber
- 1 lemon (peeled)
- 1 cup of water

NUTRITIONAL INFORMATION (PER SERVING):

- 60 calories
- 15g carbohydrate
- 4g fiber
- 2g protein
- Fat: 0.5g

INSTRUCTIONS:

1. Beet Preparation: Peel and cut the beet.

2. Rinse Berries: Thoroughly rinse the mixed berries.

3. Cucumber and Lemon Preparation: Peel and cut the cucumber. Lemon should be peeled.

4. Blend diced beet, mixed berries, cucumber, peeled lemon, and water in a blender.

5. Blend Until Smooth: Blend until the mixture is smooth.

6. Optional: Strain the juice to get a smoother texture.

7. Pour this detoxifying beet berry combination into a glass and enjoy.

CARROT GINGER INFUSION FOR CLEANSING

- Time to Prepare: 5 minutes
- 1 serving size
- Time to cook: 0 minutes

INGREDIENTS:

- 2 medium peeled and sliced carrots
- 1 inch peeled ginger
- 1/2 peeled and segmented orange
- 1 lime (juiced)
- 1 cup of water

NUTRITIONAL INFORMATION (PER SERVING):

- 50 calories
- 12g carbohydrate
- 3g fiber
- 1g protein
- Fat: 0.5g

INSTRUCTIONS:

1. Carrots should be peeled and chopped.
2. Peel and finely cut the ginger.
3. Prepare the orange and lime by peeling and segmenting the orange. Make lime juice.
4. In a blender, add the carrots, ginger, orange segments, lime juice, and water.
5. Blend Until Smooth: Blend until the mixture is smooth.
6. Optional: Strain the juice to get a smoother texture.
7. Pour into a glass and enjoy this revitalizing carrot ginger infusion.

DETOX SPLASH WITH MINTY MELON

- Time to Prepare: 8 minutes
- 1 serving size
- Time to cook: 0 minutes

INGREDIENTS:

- 1 cup sliced watermelon
- 1/2 peeled and sliced cucumber
- a few fresh mint leaves
- 1 lime (juiced)
- 1 cup of water

NUTRITIONAL INFORMATION (PER SERVING):

- 40 calories
- 10g carbohydrate
- 2g fiber
- 1g protein
- Fat: 0.5g

INSTRUCTIONS:

1. Watermelon Dice: Cut watermelon into cubes.
2. Cucumber Preparation: Peel and cut cucumber.
3. Mint Preparation: Wash and dry fresh mint leaves.
4. Lime Juice: Extract the juice from the lime.
5. Blend together sliced watermelon, chopped cucumber, fresh mint leaves, lime juice, and water in a blender.
6. Blend Until Smooth: Blend until the mixture is smooth.
7. Pour this minty melon detox splash into a glass and enjoy.

JUICE OF PINEAPPLE AND PAPAYA

- Time to Prepare: 7 minutes
- 1 serving size
- Time to cook: 0 minutes

INGREDIENTS:

- 1 cup diced fresh pineapple
- 1/2 cup sliced ripe papaya
- 1 lemon (peeled)
- 1 tablespoon turmeric powder
- 1 cup of water

NUTRITIONAL INFORMATION (PER SERVING):

- 60 calories
- 15g carbohydrate
- 3g fiber
- 1g protein
- Fat: 0.5g

INSTRUCTIONS:

1. Pineapple and Papaya Cubes: Cut fresh pineapple and ripe papaya into cubes.
2. Lemon Preparation: Peel the lemon.
3. Turmeric Powder: Mix with turmeric powder.
4. Blend chopped pineapple, diced papaya, peeled lemon, turmeric powder, and water in a blender.
5. Blend Until Smooth: Blend until the mixture is smooth.
6. Pour this pineapple papaya purifier juice into a glass and enjoy.

DETOX ELIXIR WITH BLUEBERRIES AND BASIL

- Time to Prepare: 6 minutes
- 1 serving size
- Time to cook: 0 minutes

- 1 cup fresh blueberries
- a few fresh basil leaves
- 1/2 peeled and sliced cucumber
- 1 lemon (peeled)
- 1 cup of water

NUTRITIONAL INFORMATION (PER SERVING):

- 45 calories
- 11g carbohydrate
- 3g fiber
- 1g protein
- Fat: 0.5g

INSTRUCTIONS:

1. Blueberries should be well rinsed.
2. Basil Preparation: Wash and prepare fresh basil leaves.
3. Cucumber and Lemon Preparation: Peel and cut the cucumber. Lemon should be peeled.
4. Rinse blueberries, fresh basil leaves, diced cucumber, peeled lemon, and water in a blender.
5. Blend Until Smooth: Blend until the mixture is smooth.
6. Optional: Strain the juice to get a smoother texture.
7. Pour this blueberry basil detox elixir into a glass and enjoy.

TWIST OF TROPICAL TURMERIC

- Time to Prepare: 7 minutes
- 1 serving size
- Time to cook: 0 minutes

INGREDIENTS:

- 1-pound pineapple chunks
- half a cup mango chunks
- 1 tablespoon turmeric powder
- 1 lemon (juiced)
- 1-liter coconut water

NUTRITIONAL INFORMATION (PER SERVING):

- 70 calories
- 18g carbohydrate
- 2g fiber
- 1g protein
- Fat: 0.5g

INSTRUCTIONS:

1. Pineapple and Mango Preparation: Cut pineapple and mango into pieces.
2. Turmeric Powder: Mix with turmeric powder.
3. Lemon Juice: Extract the juice from the lemon.

4. Blend pineapple chunks, mango chunks, turmeric powder, lemon juice, and coconut water in a blender.

5. Blend Until Smooth: Blend until the mixture is smooth.

6. Pour into a glass and serve with a tropical turmeric twist.

CLEANSE WITH ROSEMARY AND CITRUS

- Time to Prepare: 8 minutes
- 1 serving size
- Time to cook: 0 minutes

INGREDIENTS:

- 1 peeled and segmented orange
- 1/2 peeled and sliced grapefruit
- 1 fresh rosemary sprig
- 1 lemon (peeled)
- 1 cup of water

NUTRITIONAL INFORMATION (PER SERVING):

- 50 calories
- 12g carbohydrate
- 3g fiber
- 1g protein
- Fat: 0.5g

INSTRUCTIONS:

- Citrus preparation: Peel and section orange and grapefruit.
- Rosemary: Add a sprig of fresh rosemary.
- Lemon Preparation: Peel the lemon.
- Blend the orange and grapefruit segments, fresh rosemary, peeled lemon, and water in a blender.
- Blend Until Smooth: Blend until the mixture is smooth.
- Optional: Strain the juice to get a smoother texture.
- Pour this delightful rosemary citrus cleanse into a glass and enjoy.

CUCUMBER MINT DETOX DRINK

- Time to Prepare: 6 minutes
- 1 serving size
- Time to cook: 0 minutes

INGREDIENTS:

- 1/2 peeled and sliced cucumber
- a few fresh mint leaves
- 1 lime (juiced)
- 1 tsp. chia seeds
- 1 cup of water

- 30 calories
- 7g carbohydrate
- 2g fiber
- 1g protein
- Fat: 0.5g

INSTRUCTIONS:

1. Cucumber Preparation: Peel and cut cucumber.
2. Mint Preparation: Wash and dry fresh mint leaves.
3. Lime Juice: Extract the juice from the lime.
4. Include Chia Seeds: Chia seeds may be used for texture.
5. Blend diced cucumber, fresh mint leaves, lime juice, chia seeds, and water in a blender.
6. Blend Until Smooth: Blend until the mixture is smooth.
7. Pour this cucumber mint detox splash into a glass and enjoy.

DANDELION GREEN ELIXIR FOR DETOXIFICATION

- Time to Prepare: 7 minutes
- 1 serving size
- Time to cook: 0 minutes

INGREDIENTS:

- 1 cup washed dandelion greens
- 1/2 peeled and sliced cucumber
- 1 green apple, cored and diced
- 1 lemon (peeled)
- 1-liter coconut water

NUTRITIONAL INFORMATION (PER SERVING):

- 45 calories
- 11g carbohydrate
- 3g fiber
- 2g protein
- Fat: 0.5g

INSTRUCTIONS:

1. Dandelion Greens: Thoroughly wash dandelion greens.
2. Cucumber and Apple Preparation: Peel and cut cucumber. Remove the core and cut the green apple.
3. Lemon Preparation: Peel the lemon.
4. Blend washed dandelion greens, diced cucumber, chopped green apple,

peeled lemon, and coconut water in a blender.

5. Blend Until Smooth: Blend until the mixture is smooth.

6. Optional: Strain the elixir to get a smoother texture.

7. Pour this cleansing dandelion green elixir into a glass and drink.

DETOX WITH SPICY GINGER LEMONADE

- Time to Prepare: 6 minutes
- 1 serving size
- Time to cook: 0 minutes

INGREDIENTS:

- 1 lemon (peeled)
- 1 inch peeled ginger
- 1 tsp cayenne pepper
- 1 teaspoon (optional) honey
- 1 cup of water

NUTRITIONAL INFORMATION (PER SERVING):

- 20 calories
- 6g carbohydrate
- 1g fiber
- 0.5g protein
- Fat: 0.5g

INSTRUCTIONS:

1. Lemon and Ginger Preparation: Peel the lemon and ginger.

2. Cayenne Pepper: Mix in a pinch of cayenne pepper.

3. Optional Sweetener: If desired, add honey.

4. Blend the peeled lemon, peeled ginger, cayenne pepper, honey, and water in a blender.

5. Blend Until Smooth: Blend until the mixture is smooth.

6. Pour this spicy ginger lemonade detox into a glass and enjoy.

CLASSIC CARROT-CELERY REFRESHER

- Preparation Time: 5 minutes
- Cooking Time: 0 minutes
- Serving Size: 1

INGREDIENTS:

- 3 big peeled and chopped carrots 3 celery stalks cut 1/2 lemon, peeled 1 cup water

NUTRITIONAL INFORMATION (PER SERVING):

- 50 calories
- 12g carbohydrate
- 3g fiber
- 2g protein
- Fat: 0.5g

INSTRUCTIONS:

1. Prepare the carrots and celery as follows: Carrots should be peeled and chopped. Chop the celery.
2. Prepare the Lemon: Remove the peel from the lemon.
3. Blend: In a blender, add the carrots, celery, lemon peel, and water.
4. Blend until completely smooth: Blend until a smooth texture is produced.
5. Optional: Strain the juice to get a smoother texture.
6. Pour into a glass and enjoy this traditional carrot-celery refreshment.

GREEN SPINACH-PARSLEY MEDLEY

- Time to Prepare: 7 minutes
- 1 serving size
- Time to cook: 0 minutes

INGREDIENTS:

- 1 cup freshly chopped spinach leaves
- a sprig of fresh parsley
- 1/2 peeled and sliced cucumber
- 1 green apple, cored and diced
- 1 cup of water

NUTRITIONAL INFORMATION (PER SERVING):

- 40 calories
- 10g carbohydrate
- 3g fiber
- 1g protein
- Fat: 0.5g

1. Prepare the spinach and parsley as follows: Fresh spinach and parsley should be washed.
2. Cucumber and Apple Preparation: Cucumber should be peeled and chopped. Remove the core and cut the green apple.
3. Blend together fresh spinach leaves, parsley, cucumber, green apple, and water in a blender.
4. Blend until completely smooth: Blend until a smooth texture is produced.
5. Pour this green spinach-parsley combination into a glass and serve.

BEETROOT-CARROT VITALITY BLEND

- Preparation Time: 6 Minutes
- Cooking Time: 0 minutes
- Serving Size: 1

INGREDIENTS:

- 1 medium-sized peeled and sliced beet
- 2 medium-sized peeled and sliced carrots 1/2 orange, peeled and segments
- 1 cup water 1/2 lemon, peeled

NUTRITIONAL INFORMATION (PER SERVING):

- 60 calories
- 15g carbohydrate
- 4g fiber
- 2g protein
- Fat: 0.5g

INSTRUCTIONS:

1. Prepare the beets and carrots as follows: Peel and dice the beets and carrots.
2. Peel the orange and lemon and set aside.
3. Blend: In a blender, add the diced beet, carrots, orange segments, lemon segments, and water.
4. Blend until completely smooth: Blend until a smooth texture is produced.
5. Optional: Strain the juice to get a smoother texture.
6. Pour this beetroot-carrot vitality combination into a glass and enjoy.

GARDEN TOMATO-CUCUMBER INFUSION

- Time to Prepare: 7 minutes
- 1 serving size
- Time to cook: 0 minutes

INGREDIENTS:

- 2 big tomatoes, peeled and diced 1/2 cucumber, peeled and sliced
- a few fresh basil leaves
- 1 cup water 1/2 lemon, juiced

NUTRITIONAL INFORMATION (PER SERVING):

- 35 calories
- 8g carbohydrate
- 2g fiber
- 1g protein
- Fat: 0.5g

INSTRUCTIONS:

1. Tomatoes and cucumber should be prepared as follows: Wash and cut the tomatoes. Cucumber should be peeled and chopped.
2. Prepare the basil: Fresh basil leaves should be washed and prepared.
3. Lemon Juice: Extract the juice from the lemon.
4. Blend chopped tomatoes, cucumber, fresh basil leaves, lemon juice, and water in a blender.
5. Blend until completely smooth: Blend until a smooth texture is produced.
6. Pour this tomato-cucumber garden infusion into a glass and enjoy.

SPICY KALE-TURMERIC

- Time to Prepare: 6 minutes
- Cooking Time: 0 minutes
- Serving Size: 1

INGREDIENTS:

- 1 cup kale leaves (with stems removed)
- 1/2 peeled and sliced cucumber
- 1 lemon (peeled)
- 1 tablespoon turmeric powder
- 1 tsp cayenne pepper
- 1 cup of water

NUTRITIONAL INFORMATION (PER SERVING):

- 40 calories
- 9g Carbohydrates
- 3g fiber
- 2g protein
- Fat: 0.5g

1. Remove the Kale Stems: Remove the stems from the kale leaves.

2. Cucumber with Lemon Preparation: Cucumber should be peeled and chopped. Lemon should be peeled.

3. Turmeric with cayenne pepper: Add a pinch of cayenne pepper and turmeric powder.

4. Blend kale leaves (stems removed), diced cucumber, peeled lemon, turmeric powder, cayenne pepper, and water in a blender.

5. Blend until completely smooth: Blend until a smooth texture is produced.

6. Pour this spicy kale-turmeric jolt into a glass and enjoy.

ZESTY BELL PEPPER-CARROT FUSION

- Time to Prepare: 7 minutes
- 1 serving size
- Time to cook: 0 minutes

INGREDIENTS:

- 1 big sliced bell pepper 2 medium-sized carrots peeled and diced
- 1/2 orange peeled and segments
- 1 cup water 1/2 lemon, peeled

NUTRITIONAL INFORMATION (PER SERVING):

- 45 calories
- 10g carbohydrate
- 3g fiber
- 2g protein
- Fat: 0.5g

INSTRUCTIONS:

1. Prepare the bell pepper and carrots as follows: Wash and cut the bell pepper. Carrots should be peeled and chopped.

2. Peel the orange and lemon and set aside.

3. Blend: In a blender, mix diced bell pepper, carrots, orange segments, lemon segments, and water.

4. Blend until completely smooth: Blend until a smooth texture is produced.

5. Optional: Strain the juice to get a smoother texture.

6. Pour this fiery bell pepper-carrot mix into a glass and enjoy.

CABBAGE-APPLE DETOX ELIXIR

INGREDIENTS:

- 1 cup shredded cabbage, 1 cup shredded carrots
- 1 green apple, cored and diced
- 1 lemon (peeled)
- 1 teaspoon grated ginger
- 1 cup of water

NUTRITIONAL INFORMATION (PER SERVING):

- 35 calories
- 8g carbohydrate
- 3g fiber
- 1g protein
- Fat: 0.5g

INSTRUCTIONS:

1. Cabbage, shredded: Finely shred the cabbage.
2. Prepare the Apple: The green apple should be peeled and chopped.
3. Lemon Preparation: Peel the lemon.
4. Ginger, grated: Include grated ginger.
5. Blend together shredded cabbage, diced green apple, peeled lemon, grated ginger, and water in a blender.
6. Blend until completely smooth: Blend until a smooth texture is produced.
7. Pour this cabbage-apple detox elixir into a glass and drink.

JUICE OF BROCCOLI AND CUCUMBER

INGREDIENTS:

- 1 cup broccoli florets, 1 cup steamed broccoli, 1 cup steamed broccoli, 1 cup
- 1/2 peeled and sliced cucumber
- a few fresh mint leaves
- 1 lemon (peeled)
- 1 cup of water

NUTRITIONAL INFORMATION (PER SERVING):

- 40 calories
- 9g Carbohydrates
- 3g fiber
- 2g protein
- Fat: 0.5g

INSTRUCTIONS:

1. Trim and wash broccoli florets before cooking.

2. Cucumber Preparation: Peel and cut cucumber.

3. Mint Preparation: Wash and dry fresh mint leaves.

4. Lemon Preparation: Peel the lemon.

5. Blend broccoli florets, cucumber, fresh mint leaves, peeled lemon, and water in a blender.

6. Blend until completely smooth: Blend until a smooth texture is produced.

7. Pour this broccoli-cucumber cleansing juice into a glass and enjoy.

SWEET POTATO-SPINACH REVITALIZER

- Time to Prepare: 8 minutes
- Cooking Time: 0 minutes
- Serving Size: 1

INGREDIENTS:

- 1 medium-sized peeled and sliced sweet potato
- 1 cup spinach leaves, fresh
- 1/2 peeled and segmented orange
- 1 lemon (peeled)
- 1 cup of water

NUTRITIONAL INFORMATION (PER SERVING):

- 60 calories
- 14g carbohydrate
- 4g fiber
- 2g protein
- Fat: 0.5g

INSTRUCTIONS:

- Make the Sweet Potato: The sweet potato should be peeled and chopped.
- Wash Spinach: Thoroughly wash fresh spinach leaves.
- Peel the orange and lemon and set aside.
- Blend diced sweet potato, fresh spinach leaves, peeled orange segments, peeled lemon, and water in a blender.
- Blend until completely smooth: Blend until a smooth texture is produced.
- Optional: Strain the juice to get a smoother texture.
- Pour this sweet potato-spinach revitalizer into a glass and enjoy.

CITRUS-CARROT ASPARAGUS SPLASH

- Time to Prepare: 7 minutes
- 1 serving size
- Time to cook: 0 minutes

INGREDIENTS:

- 1 cup trimmed and chopped asparagus
- 2 medium-sized carrots peeled and sliced
- 1/2 orange peeled and segments
- 1 cup water 1/2 lemon, peeled

NUTRITIONAL INFORMATION (PER SERVING):

- 50 calories
- 12g carbohydrate
- 4g fiber
- 2g protein
- Fat: 0.5g

INSTRUCTIONS:

1. Asparagus: Trim and cut the asparagus.
2. Carrots should be peeled and chopped.
3. Peel the orange and lemon and set aside.
4. Blend: In a blender, add chopped asparagus, carrots, orange segments, lemon segments, and water.
5. Blend until completely smooth: Blend until a smooth texture is produced.
6. Pour this asparagus-carrot citrus splash into a glass and enjoy.

RADISH-BEET BLISSFUL BLEND

- Time to Prepare: 6 minutes
- Cooking Time: 0 minutes
- Serving Size: 1

INGREDIENTS:

- 1 cup trimmed and chopped radishes
- 1 medium peeled and sliced beet 1/2 orange, peeled and segments
- 1 cup water 1/2 lemon, peeled

NUTRITIONAL INFORMATION (PER SERVING):

- 55 calories
- 13g carbohydrate
- 4g fiber
- 2g protein
- Fat: 0.5g

INSTRUCTIONS:

1. Radishes should be trimmed: Radishes should be peeled and chopped.

2. Beet Preparation: Peel and cut the beet.

3. Peel the orange and lemon and set aside.

4. Blend: Combine chopped radishes, diced beets, peeled orange segments, peeled lemon, and water in a blender.

5. Blend until completely smooth: Blend until a smooth texture is produced.

6. Optional: Strain the juice to get a smoother texture.

7. Pour this radish-beet delightful combination into a glass and enjoy.

GREEN SYMPHONY OF ZUCCHINI AND CELERY

- 1/2 zucchini, peeled and cut 3 celery stalks, chopped
- 1/2 cucumber, peeled and sliced
- a sprig of fresh parsley
- 1 cup water 1/2 lemon, peeled

- 35 calories
- 8g carbohydrate
- 3g fiber
- 1g protein
- Fat: 0.5g

1. Prepare the zucchini, celery, and cucumber as follows: Peel and cut cucumber, zucchini, and celery.

2. Parsley Preparation: Wash and prepare fresh parsley.

3. Lemon Preparation: Peel the lemon.

4. In a blender, add the diced zucchini, celery, cucumber, fresh parsley, peeled lemon, and water.

5. Blend until completely smooth: Blend until a smooth texture is produced.

6. Pour into a glass and enjoy this green symphony of zucchini and celery.

1. Q: Is juicing a healthy alternative for diabetics?

   A: Yes, juicing may be part of a diabetes-friendly diet when done with glycemic effect and portion proportions in mind.

2. Q: Which fruits are appropriate for diabetic-friendly juices?

   A: Berries, cherries, apples (in moderation), and citrus fruits are low on the glycemic index.

3. Can I use bananas in diabetic juices?

   A: Although bananas contain more sugar, they may be consumed in moderation when combined with low-glycemic fruits and vegetables.

4. Q: Are there some veggies to avoid in diabetes juices?

   A: Because starchy vegetables like potatoes and beets may affect blood sugar levels, they should be consumed in moderation.

5. Q: How much juice is safe for someone with diabetes to consume?

   A: It is critical to keep track of portion proportions. A modest portion (4-6 ounces) is a good place to start.

6. Q: Is it preferable to eat whole fruits and veggies or juice when you have diabetes?

   A: Whole fruits and vegetables include more fiber, which may aid with blood sugar stabilization. Juicing should be used to supplement a healthy diet.

7. Q: Can someone with diabetes replace meals with juicing?

   A: Juices should not be used to substitute meals. Juices may be used as a snack or as a meal replacement.

8. Q: Should I keep sweets out of diabetic juices?

   A: It is best to avoid added sweeteners. Use modest quantities of low-calorie sweeteners if sweetness is required.

9. Q: Can green juices help those who have diabetes?

   A: Green juices made from leafy greens such as spinach and kale may deliver necessary nutrients while having a lesser effect on blood sugar.

10. Q: How does fiber affect diabetic juicing?

A: Fiber slows sugar absorption, resulting in improved blood sugar regulation. Consider incorporating pulp into your juice.

11. Q: When juicing, is it important to monitor blood sugar levels more frequently?

A: It is critical to monitor blood sugar levels, particularly when introducing new foods or liquids into your diet.

12. Q: Do you have any juicing recipes for diabetic management?

A: Low-glycemic fruit and vegetable recipes, such as green vegetable juices, may be useful.

13. Q: Can juicing help persons with diabetes lose weight?

A: Juicing, when combined with a well-balanced diet, may help with weight management, which is excellent for diabetes control.

14. Q: How can I keep the sugar content of my juices under control?

A: Use low-glycemic fruits, restrict high-sugar fruits, and watch portion sizes

15. Q: Are there any juicing procedures that are specifically advised for diabetics?

A: Cold-press or masticating juicers retain more nutrients than high-speed centrifugal juicers and may be preferable.

16. Q: Can I make diabetic juice with herbs and spices?

A: Yes, plants like cilantro and spices like cinnamon may enhance taste without affecting blood sugar levels much.

17. Q: What effect does juicing have on insulin sensitivity?

A: While some research suggests eating particular juices may enhance insulin sensitivity, individual responses may differ.

18. Q: Can juicing cause hypoglycemia in diabetic patients?

A: Excessive juicing, if not balanced with other meals, might result in low blood sugar. Keep an eye on your levels on a frequent basis.

19. Q: Should I visit a healthcare professional before beginning a diabetic juicing regimen?

A: Yes, it is recommended that you speak with a healthcare physician or a dietician to verify that your juicing plan is appropriate for your unique health requirements.

20. Q: Can I make a juice out of frozen fruits and vegetables?

A: Yes, utilizing frozen veggies is a handy and nutritious choice.

21. Q: What function does hydration play in diabetes and juicing?

A: It is important to stay hydrated. Although juices might help with fluid intake, water should remain be the preferred beverage.

22. Q: Can juicing create stomach troubles in diabetics?

A: Excessive juicing might cause stomach problems. Include fiber-rich foods and think about the overall balance of your diet.

23. Q: Should I be worried about the naturally occurring sugars in fruits while juicing?

A: To reduce the influence on blood sugar, watch portion sizes and pick fruits with reduced sugar content.

24. Q: Can I solely juice non-starchy vegetables?

A: While non-starchy veggies are preferred, a variety of vegetables, including ones with modest starch, may be consumed in moderation.

25. Q: Can juicing increase energy levels in diabetics?

A well-balanced diet, including nutrient-dense juices, may help maintain energy levels.

26. Q: Are there any hazards to juicing for those with diabetes?

A: Risks include blood sugar rises if not done carefully. Regular supervision and moderation are essential.

27. Q: Can juicing affect diabetic medications?

A: It is important to notify your healthcare physician about dietary changes since medicines may need to be adjusted.

28. Q: Can juicing be used into a long-term diabetes control strategy?

A: Yes, juicing may help with long-term diabetes treatment when done correctly and as part of a healthy lifestyle.

29. Q: Can juicing lead to vitamin shortages in diabetics?

A: Preventing nutritional imbalances requires a diversified and balanced juicing strategy, as well as a varied diet.

30. Q: How can I make juicing a component of my diabetes treatment that is both sustainable and enjoyable?

A: For long-term adherence, experiment with tastes, integrate a range of fruits and vegetables, and customize recipes to your taste preferences.

Remember that individual reactions to juicing might vary, so tailor your strategy to your own health requirements and tastes. For individualized counsel, always speak with your healthcare physician or a licensed dietician.

RECIPE JOURNAL

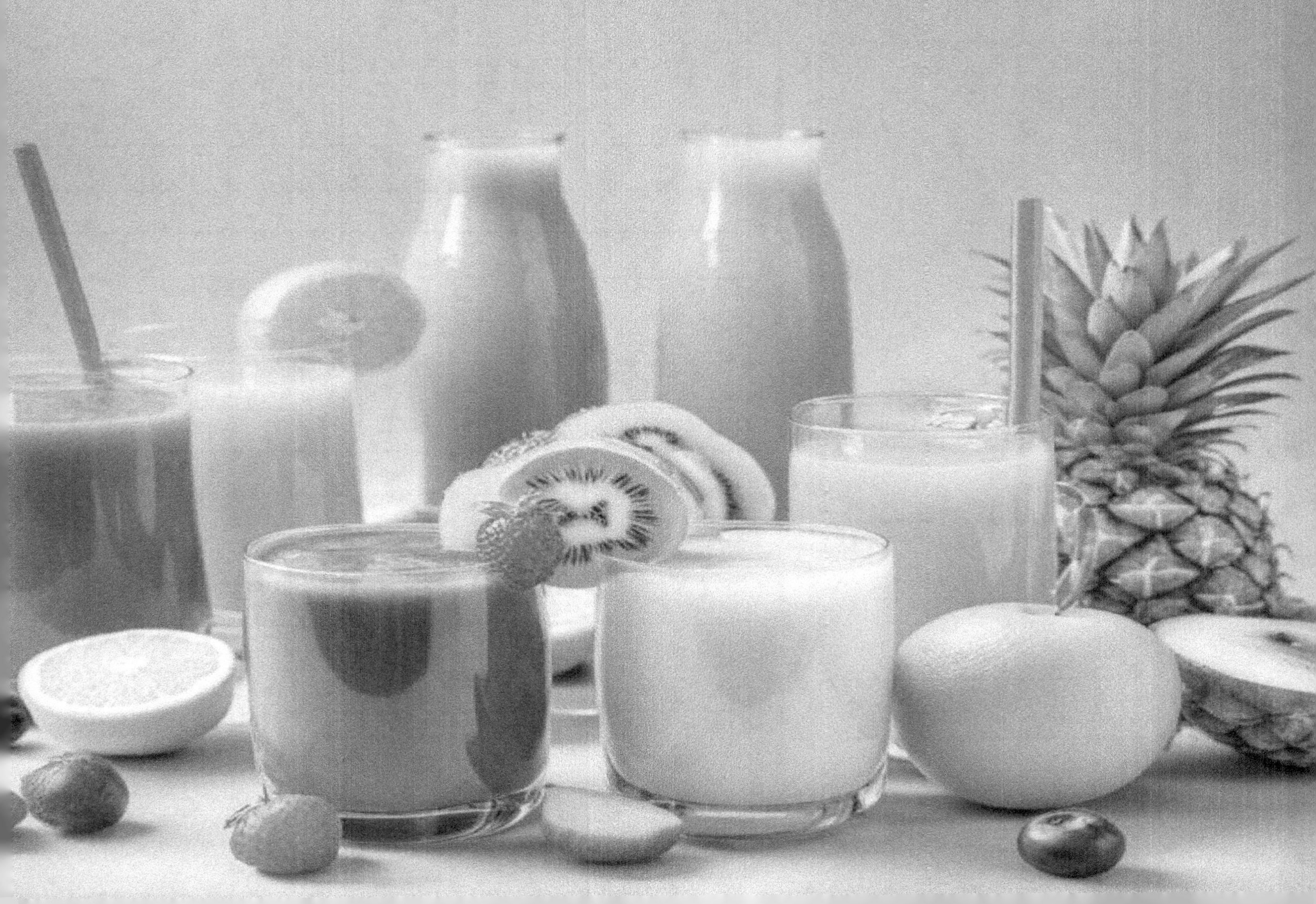

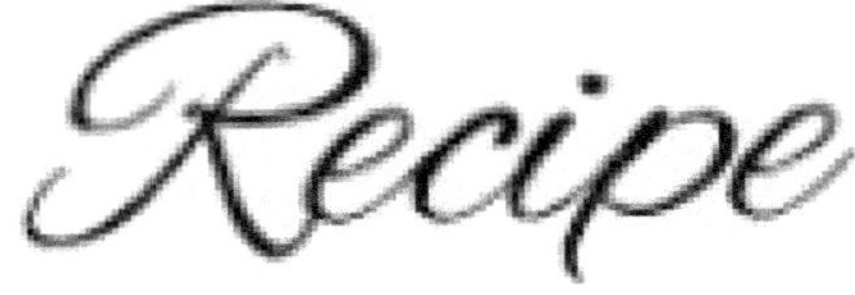

Category

Servings _________________

Prep time_________________

Cook time_________________

Review _________________

NOTES

Tools

____

____

Ingredients

Direction

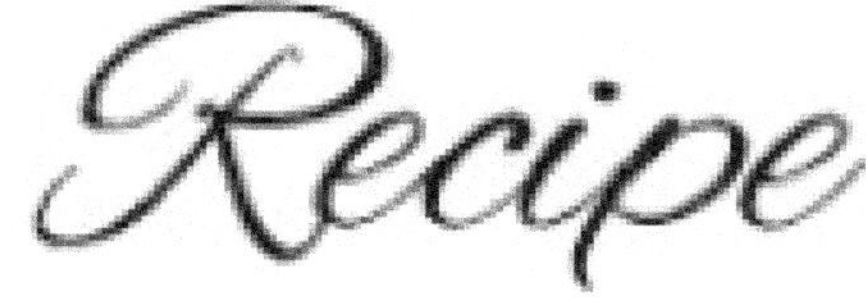

Ingredients

Category

Servings _______________

Prep time_______________

Cook time_______________

Review _______________

NOTES

Tools

____

____

Direction

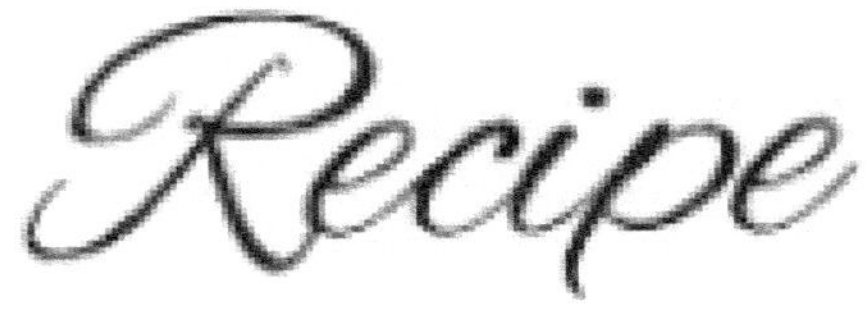

Recipe

Category

____

Servings _______________

Prep time_______________

Cook time_______________

Review _______________

NOTES

Tools

____

____

Ingredients

Direction

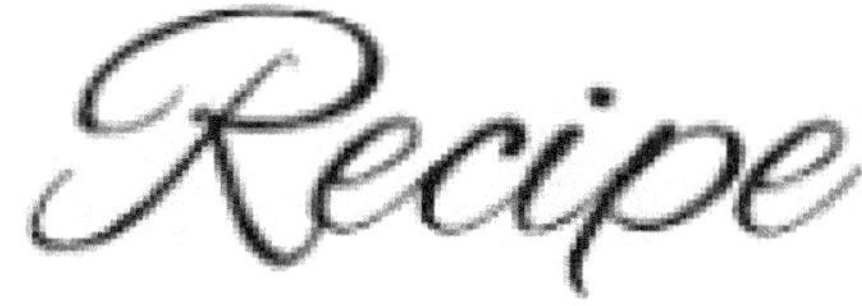

Ingredients

Category

Servings _______________

Prep time_______________

Cook time_______________

Review _______________

NOTES

Tools

Direction

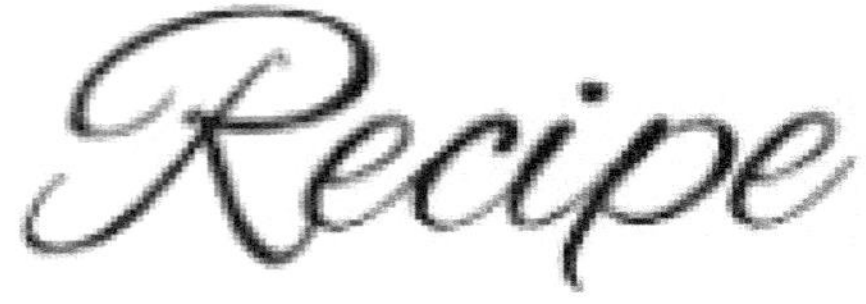

Recipe

Category

____

Servings _______________

Prep time_______________

Cook time_______________

Review _________________

NOTES

Tools

____

____

Ingredients

Direction

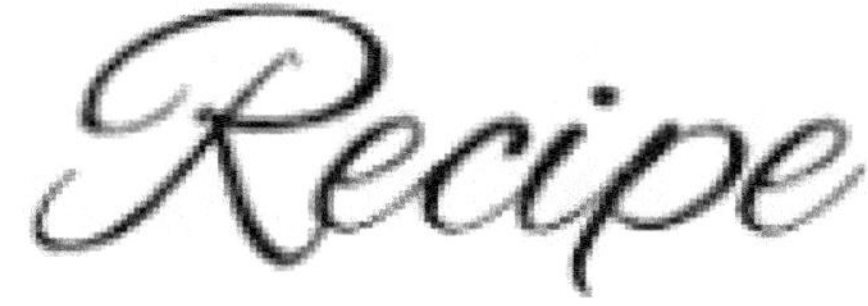

Recipe

Category

____

Servings _______________

Prep time_______________

Cook time_______________

Review _______________

NOTES

Tools

____

____

Ingredients

Direction

Recipe

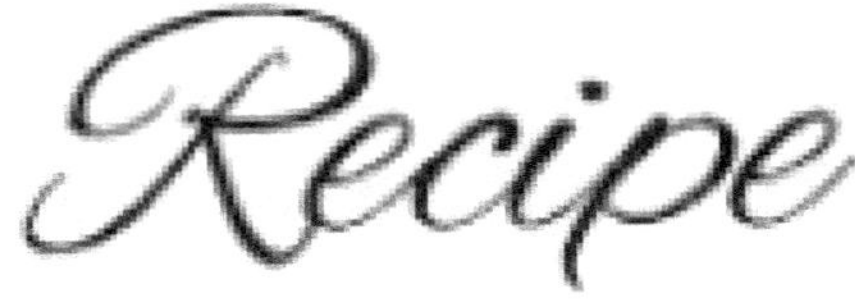

Category

____

Servings _______________

Prep time_______________

Cook time_______________

Review _________________

NOTES

Tools

____

____

Ingredients

Direction

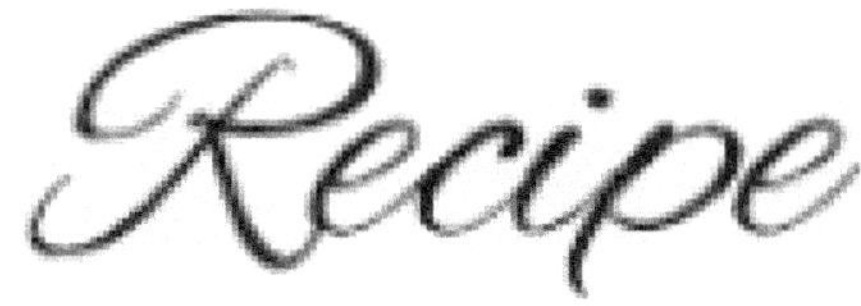

Recipe

Category

____

Servings _______________

Prep time_______________

Cook time_______________

Review _______________

NOTES

Tools

____

____

Ingredients

Direction

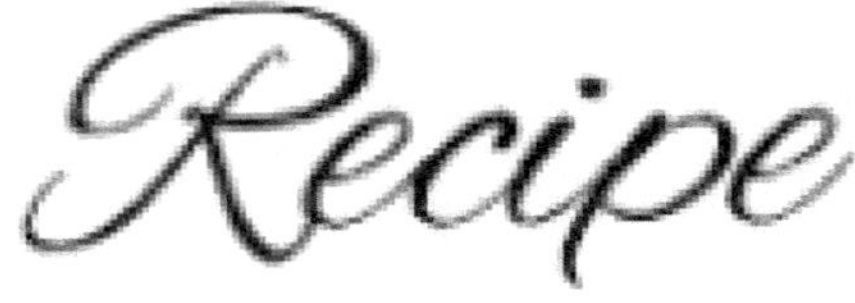

Category

____

Servings _________________

Prep time_________________

Cook time_________________

Review _________________

NOTES

Tools

____

____

Ingredients

____
____
____
____
____
____
____
____
____
____
____

Direction

____
____
____
____
____
____
____
____
____
____
____

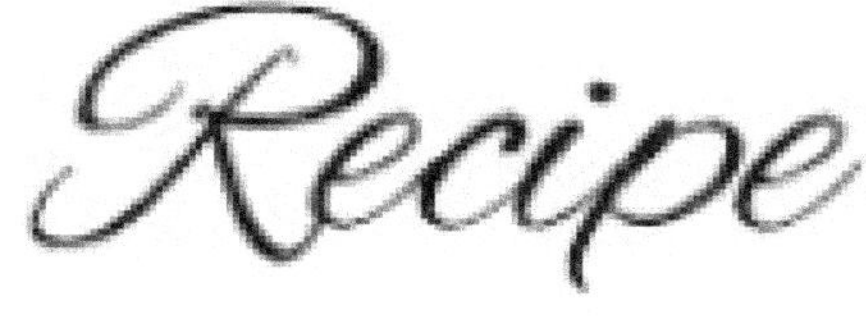

Recipe

Category

____

Servings _______________

Prep time ______________

Cook time ______________

Review ________________

NOTES

Tools

____

____

Ingredients

Direction

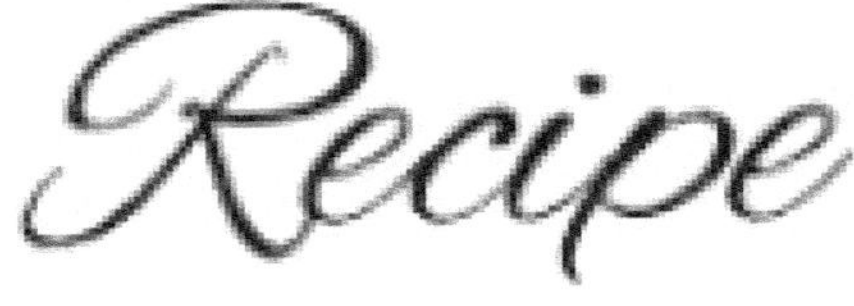

Recipe

Category

____

Servings _______________

Prep time______________

Cook time______________

Review _________________

NOTES

Tools

____

____

Ingredients

Direction

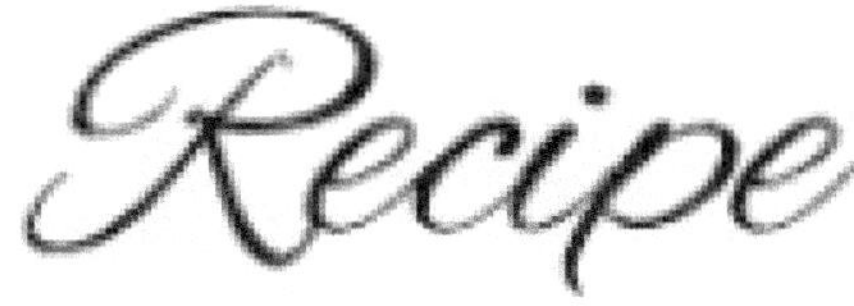

Recipe

Category

____

Servings _________________

Prep time_________________

Cook time_________________

Review _________________

NOTES

Tools

____

____

Ingredients

Direction

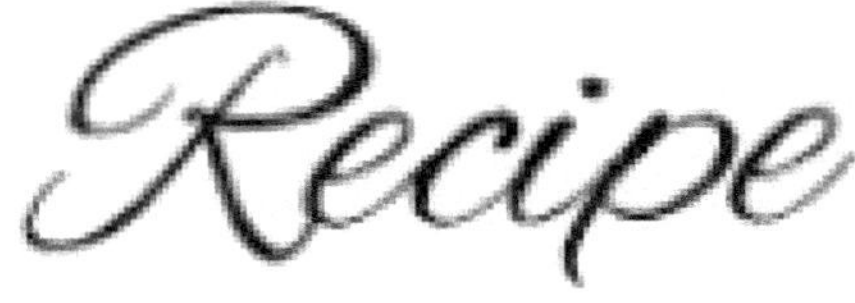

Recipe

Category

____

Servings _______________________

Prep time______________________

Cook time______________________

Review _________________________

NOTES

Tools

____

____

Ingredients

Direction

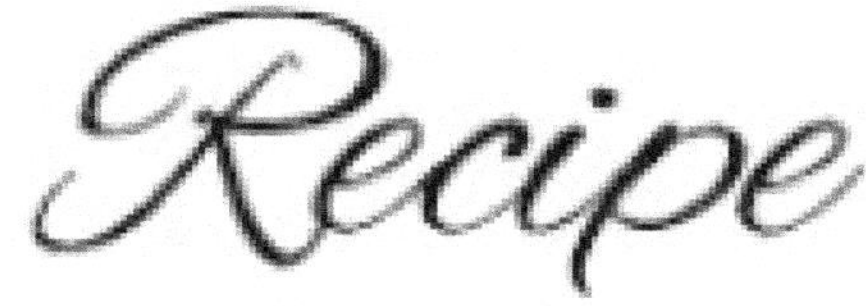

Ingredients

Category

Servings _______________

Prep time_______________

Cook time_______________

Review _______________

NOTES

Tools

Ingredients

Direction

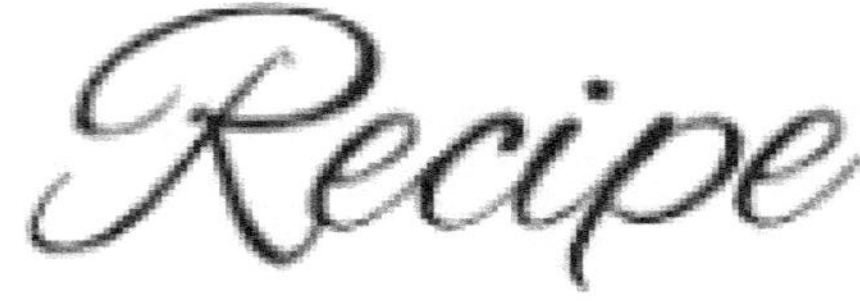

Category

Servings _______________

Prep time_______________

Cook time_______________

Review _______________

NOTES

Tools

Ingredients

Direction

Recipe

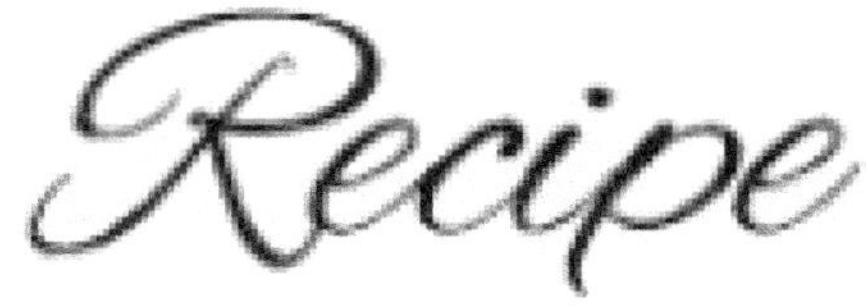

Category

____

Servings _______________

Prep time______________

Cook time______________

Review ________________

NOTES

Tools

____

____

Ingredients

Direction

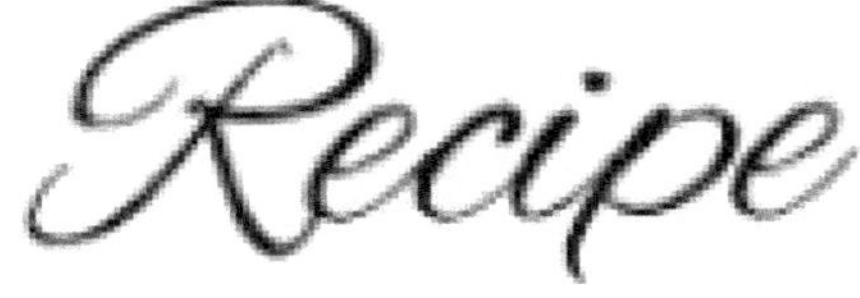

Category

Servings _________________

Prep time_________________

Cook time_________________

Review _________________

NOTES

Tools

____

____

Ingredients

Direction

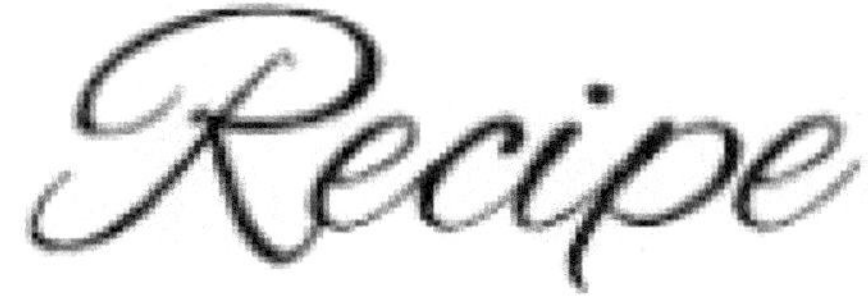

Recipe

Category

____

Servings ________________

Prep time________________

Cook time________________

Review ________________

NOTES

Tools

____

____

Ingredients

Direction

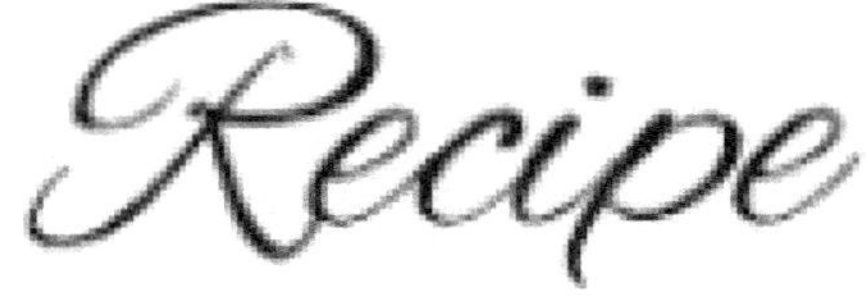

Recipe

Category

____

Servings ___________________

Prep time_________________

Cook time_________________

Review ___________________

NOTES

Tools

____

____

Ingredients

Direction

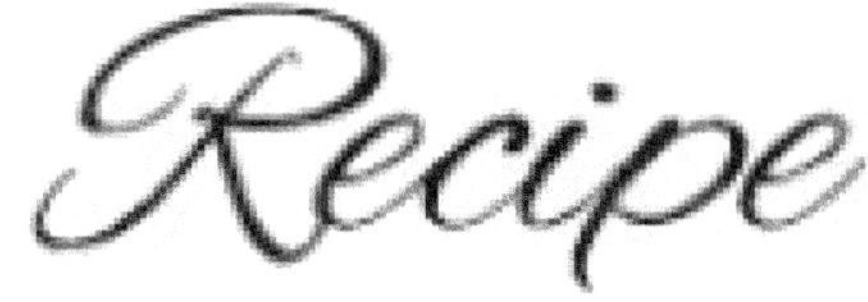

Recipe

Category

____

Servings _______________

Prep time _______________

Cook time _______________

Review _______________

NOTES

Tools

____

____

Ingredients

Direction

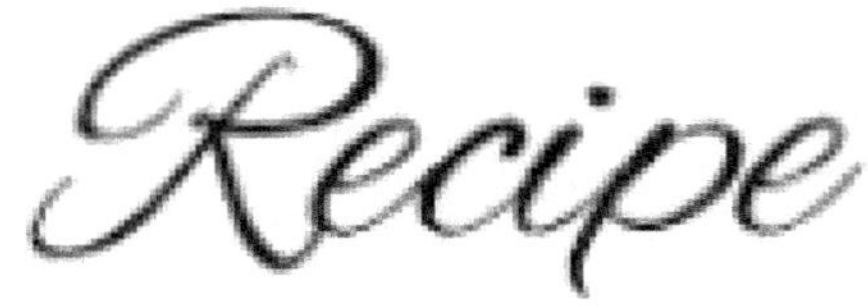

Recipe

Category

____

Servings ________________

Prep time________________

Cook time________________

Review ________________

NOTES

Tools

____

____

Ingredients

Direction

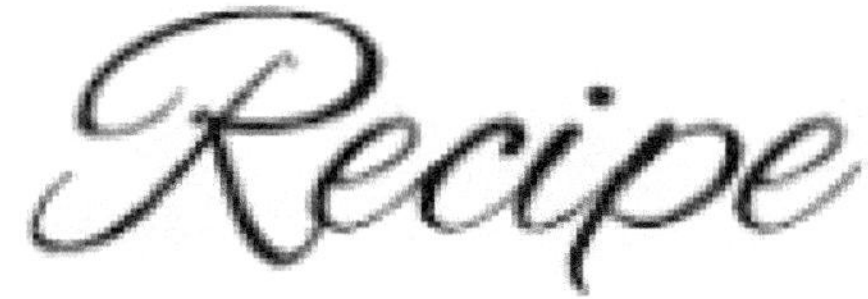

Category

Servings _______________

Prep time_______________

Cook time_______________

Review _______________

NOTES

Tools

____

Ingredients

Direction

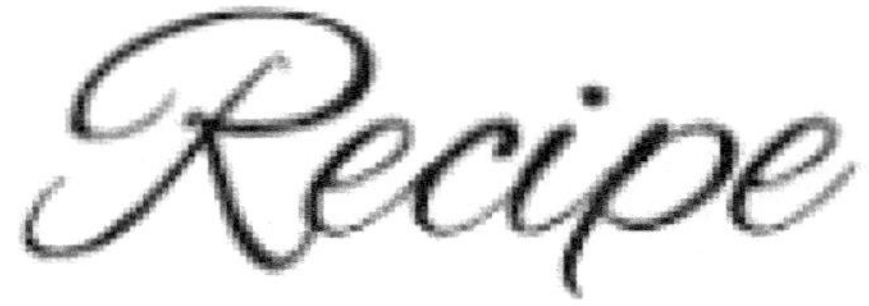

Recipe

Category

____

Servings ________________

Prep time________________

Cook time________________

Review _________________

NOTES

Tools

____

____

Ingredients

Direction

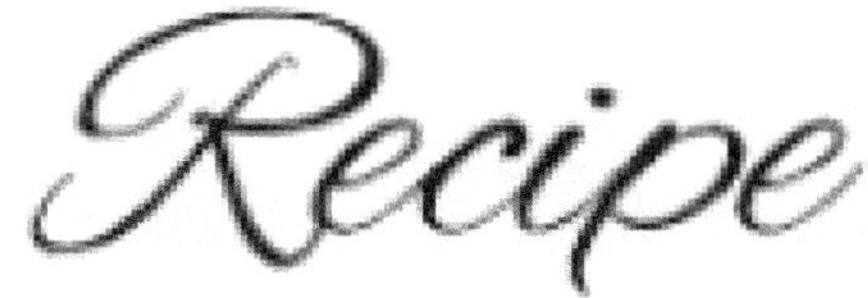

Recipe

Category

____

Servings ___________________

Prep time___________________

Cook time___________________

Review ____________________

NOTES

Tools

____

____

Ingredients

Direction

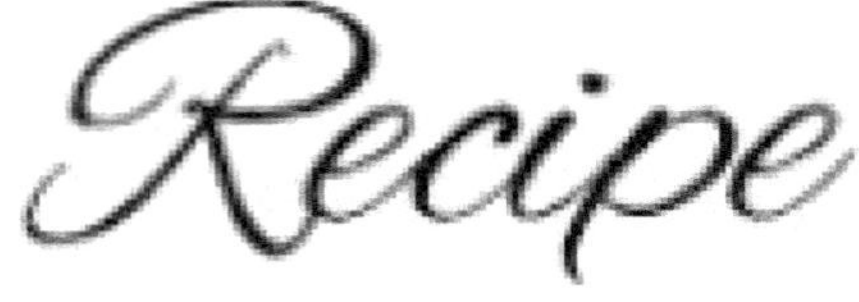

Recipe

Category

____

Servings _________________

Prep time_________________

Cook time_________________

Review _________________

NOTES

Tools

____

____

Ingredients

Direction

Recipe

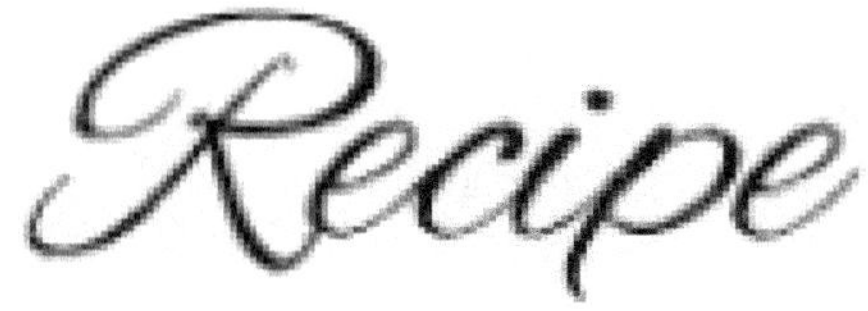

Category

____

Servings _______________

Prep time_______________

Cook time_______________

Review _________________

NOTES

Tools

____

____

Ingredients

Direction

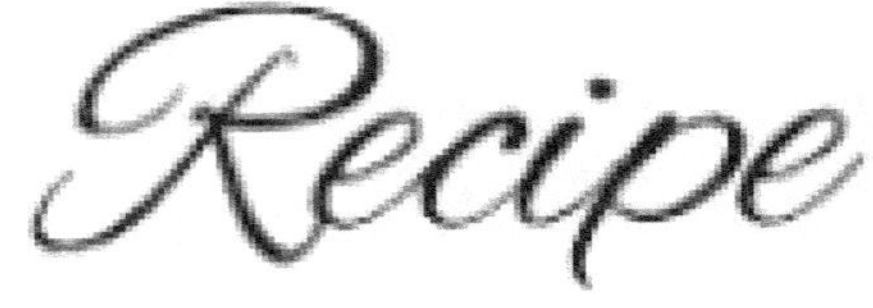

Recipe

Category

____

Servings ________________

Prep time________________

Cook time________________

Review ________________

NOTES

Tools

____

____

Ingredients

Direction

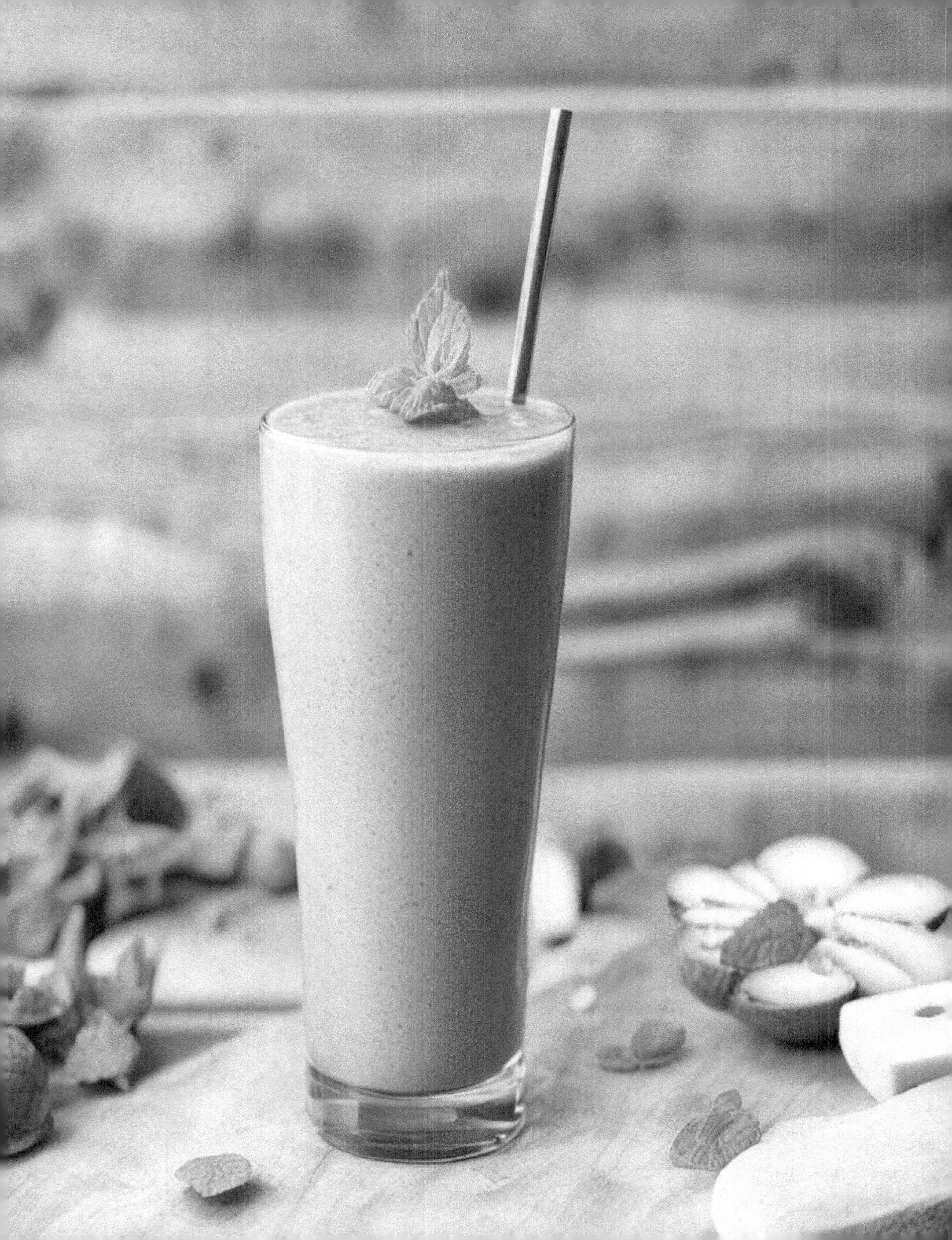

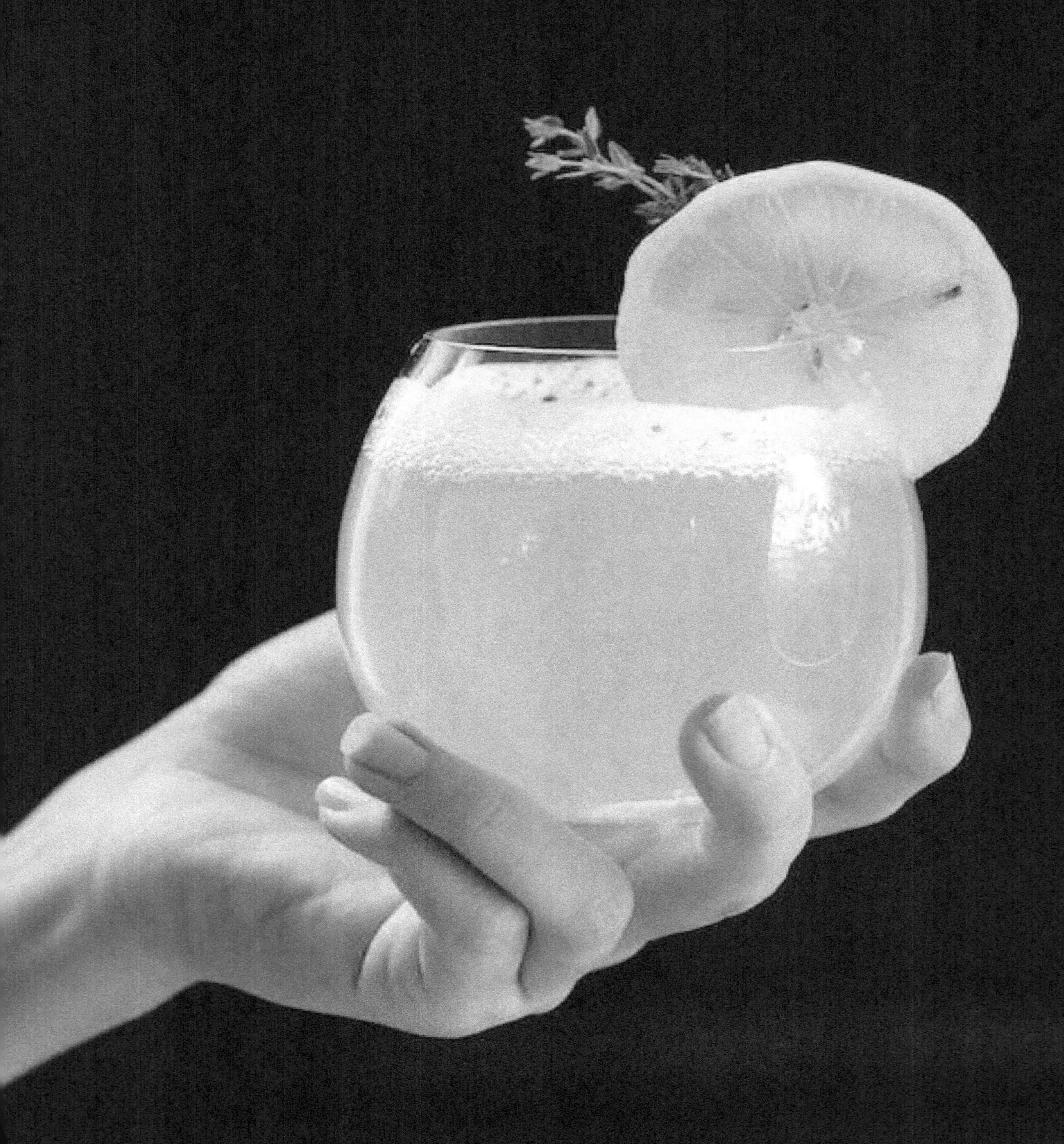